T0251274

Decade of the Plague:
The Sociopsychological
Ramifications of STD

Decade of the Plague: The Sociopsychological Ramifications of STD

Margaret Rodway
Marianne Wright
Editors

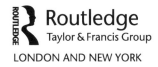

Routledge
Taylor & Francis Group

LONDON AND NEW YORK

First published 1988 by Harrington Park Press, Inc.

2 Park Square, Milton Park, Abingdon, Oxfordshire OX14 4RN
605 Third Avenue, New York, NY 10017

Routledge is an imprint of the Taylor & Francis Group, an informa business

First issued in paperback 2020

Copyright © 1988 Taylor & Francis

All rights reserved. No part of this book may be reprinted or reproduced or utilised in
any form or by any electronic, mechanical, or other means, now known or hereafter
invented, including photocopying and recording, or in any information storage or
retrieval system, without permission in writing from the publishers.

Notice:
Product or corporate names may be trademarks or registered trademarks, and are
used only for identification and explanation without intent to infringe.

Decade of the Plague: The Sociopsychological Ramifications of STD was originally published as
Journal of Social Work & Human Sexuality, Volume 6, Number 2 1988.

Cover design by Marshall Andrews.

Library of Congress Cataloging-in-Publication Data

Decade of the plague.

    "Originally published as Journal of social work and human sexuality, volume 6, number
2, 1988"—T.p. verso.
    Includes bibliographies.
    1. Sexually transmitted diseases—Social aspects. 2. Sexually transmitted
diseases—Psychological aspects. 3. Medical social work. I. Rodway, Margaret. II. Wright,
Marianne. III. Journal of social work & human sexuality.
RA644.V4D43   1988   362.1'96951   88-2271

ISBN 978-0-918393-53-1 (pbk)

CONTENTS

ABOUT THE EDITORS

Margaret Rodway, PhD, is a Professor in the Faculty of Social Welfare, The University of Calgary, where she teaches clinical social work practice and research. For the past ten years, she has been a part-time staff member and consultant to the Calgary Family Service Bureau where much of her practice is involved with sexuality issues. She has co-authored a book on dimensions of homosexuality and has also written numerous articles relating to social work practice, education, family and marital therapy and health care.

Marianne Wright, BA, BSW, MA, RSW, is a social worker in private practice in Edmonton, Alberta. She is also a part-time instructor in the Social Service Worker Program, Grant MacEwan Community College in Edmonton. She has been involved in counselling individuals with Sexually Transmitted Diseases since 1974. As part of her contract with the STD clinic in Edmonton, she has also participated in educational aspects of STD through various lectures and seminars she has conducted. She served as editor of the Proceedings of the First Family Planning Conference in Alberta. She has been in social work practice in the United States, Eastern and Western Canada for over twenty years.

Contributors

Gilbert J. Botvin, PhD, Associate Professor, Department of Psychiatry and Public Health, Cornell University Medical College, New York, New York.

Allan M. Brandt, Assistant Professor of the History of Medicine and Science, Department of Social Medicine and Health Policy, Harvard Medical School, Boston, Massachusetts.

Carole P. Christensen, DEd, Associate Professor, School of Social Work, McGill University, Montreal, Quebec.

Clarence Crossman, MDiv, Pastor, Metropolitan Community Church, London, Ontario.

June G. Hopps, PhD, Dean, Graduate School of Social Work, Boston College, Chestnut Hill, Massachusetts.

Tatiana Kitsikis, BA, MSW, Graduate Student, School of Social Work, McGill University, Montreal, Quebec.

Marian S. Krauskopf, MS, Lecturer, School of Social Work, Columbia University, New York, New York.

Constance Lindemann, DPH, Assistant Professor of Social Work and Women's Studies, School of Social Work, University of Oklahoma, Norman, Oklahoma.

John R. Moore, PhD, Lecturer, Department of Health Education, Southern Illinois University, Carbondale, Illinois.

Mario A. Orlandi, PhD, Chief, Division of Health Promotion Research, American Health Foundation, New York, New York.

Luis Palacios-Jimenez, ACSW, Co-Director, Chelsea Psychotherapy Associates, New York, New York.

Gillian Piper, BScN, Education Consultant, Sexually Transmitted Disease Control, Edmonton, Alberta.

Gerald E. Plum, PhD, Associate Professor, School of Social Work, King's College, University of Western Ontario, London, Ontario.

Barbara Romanowski, MD, Director, Sexually Transmitted Disease Control, Edmonton, Alberta.

William S. Rowe, DSW, Associate Professor, School of Social Work, King's College, University of Western Ontario, London, Ontario.

Michael Shernoff, ACSW, Co-Director, Chelsea Psychotherapy Associates, New York, New York.

Robert F. Schilling II, PhD, Assistant Professor, School of Social Work, Columbia University, New York, New York.

Steven P. Schinke, PhD, Professor, School of Social Work, Columbia University, New York, New York.

Leon F. Williams, PhD, Associate Professor, Graduate School of Social Work, Boston College, Chestnut Hill, Massachusetts.

Acknowledgements

It is with gratitude that we acknowledge the assistance of those who helped make this volume possible. We thank David A. Shore for providing the impetus for this special issue and for his helpful advice and encouragement.

The contributors to this volume, most of whom were distant in miles during the process of publication are to be commended for their enthusiasm and wisdom. As editors we were also subject to this spatial distance, but in spite of the logistical difficulties this created, we experienced much pleasure at being able to work together on the project.

Maureen Weir deserves special thanks for her skilled participation in the preparation of the manuscripts. Finally we would like to acknowledge our families and social networks for their caring and support.

Introduction

Margaret Rodway
Marianne Wright

Sexually transmitted diseases (STD) have probably been with us since the beginning of time, yet they continue to threaten our emotional and physical health and indeed our very lives. Recent media attention on herpes and now Acquired Immunodeficiency Syndrome (AIDS) have brought to our awareness the possible devastation caused by these diseases since both are at the present time incurable. Accurate statistics on herpes are difficult to obtain because in many provinces and states it is not classified as a notifiable disease. Estimates of the incidence of herpes in the United States indicate 20 million cases (Drob and Bernard, 1986) and Canadian estimates run as high as 50,000 annually (Lawlee, 1982). Although we now have more information concerning AIDS and its transmission, much of the disease remains a mystery. We still have no accurate numbers for the percentage of Human Immunodeficiency Virus (HIV) positives that will develop AIDS related complex (ARC) and AIDS. Estimates have ranged between 30 to 100%. We do know that there were 37,386 reported cases of AIDS in the United States in 1987 (U.S. Department of Health & Human Services) and 1,116 in Canada (National AIDS Centre, 1987). However, the number of HIV positive could be ten times greater than these numbers.

Although attention has been primarily focused on herpes and AIDS, they are not the only STD. While the others are curable, they too can have devastating results. Statistics confirm their epidemic proportions. In the United States in 1986, there were 67,929 cases of syphilis and 896,383 cases of gonorrhea totaling 964,312 cases of STD (U.S. Department of Health & Human Services, 1987). In

© 1988 by The Haworth Press, Inc. All rights reserved.

Canada in 1985, the most recent date for which statistics are available, there were 43,348 reported cases of STD accounting for 56% of all notifiable diseases. Of these 40,741 were gonorrhea and 2,007 were syphilis (Health and Welfare Canada, 1985). Although accurate statistics for chlamydia are just now being kept, it is estimated that for every case of gonorrhea, there are 1.5 cases of chlamydia (Alberta Social Services and Community Health, 1985).

The effects of these diseases are desolating. Beyond the almost certain death which AIDS now brings, other STD have frightening potential consequences. There is now an awareness that there may be a higher incidence of cervical cancer of women with genital herpes and that infants born during a herpes outbreak suffer a higher incidence of morbidity and death. Gonorrhea can result in sterility and chlamydia can cause both blindness and pneumonia in infants and possible death from ectopic pregnancy as well as sterility in women. Untreated syphilis can result in heart problems, insanity and eventual death and can also cause diseases in newborns.

Public response to the emergence of AIDS in particular has been one of shock, fear and disbelief, coming as it has at a time when epidemic diseases were believed to have been brought under control. There has been a strong tendency, because this disease has thus far gone beyond society's control, to treat its victims and others suspected of carrying the disease with unrestrained callousness and hostility (Goudsblom, 1986). The generally negative public attitude towards AIDS victims, their partners and families and those who are in high risk groups has served to exacerbate latent anxiety and suffering already experienced by these individuals.

No diseases evoke such strong emotional reactions as STD. Its victims are living proof that we cannot ignore our sexual behavior. They also have ramifications on relationships with others. Marriages have dissolved over the evidence of infidelity by one of the partners contracting an STD and many single people are refusing sexual involvement. Slowly as it touches more and more aspects of everyday life, AIDS in particular may transform Western society.

Medically, STD provide an almost insurmountable challenge for treatment and cure. For example, millions of dollars have been spent in research on AIDS but the outlook for a cure is not yet hopeful. STD provide a challenge as well for the other helping professionals. Carlton and Mayes (1982) have pointed out that major changes in the approaches taken will be required to meet this challenge. There has been little time for education and debate on the impact of the two non-curable STD, herpes and AIDS. Still, in the immediate future, education, not medicine may well be the single most important weapon in stemming their spread. Social work in particular has a crucial role to play in this educative function.

Similarly in terms of work with those who are already victims of the disease or closely connected to them, our profession can provide the kind of direct service which can greatly alleviate their distress. There is also an advocacy role necessary for social work to assume in terms of assuring equal and non-prejudicial treatment for all who are afflicted either directly or indirectly by STD.

This issue addresses some of the sociopsychological counseling and educative dimensions which need to be taken into account if changes in our approaches to the social problems inherent in STD are to be made.

The articles in this edition have been divided into three main and one concluding section. The first of these provides medical, social and psychological perspectives on STD. More specifically Barbara Romanowski and Gillian Piper describe the most common STD in order to provide some necessary medical information for helping professionals so that appropriate guidance and support can be given to the client/patient with an STD. Leon Williams and June Hopps illuminate some of the issues created by AIDS for minorities in order to broaden the scope of the debate relative to the policy and service delivery problems caused by the AIDS epidemic. They also make a case for an appropriate social work response to this case. Finally, the editors of this issue present the findings of their study on clients who attended an STD clinic. Their results indicate that for some individuals, STD are a symptom of stress and distress in their lives.

The second section is directed toward aspects of counseling clients with STD. Constance Lindemann views the disclosure of STD to sexual partners as an important issue in their control. She outlines the significant role which social workers can play in facilitating the disclosure of STD and identifies a number of psychosocial factors that may contribute to the difficulty individuals often experience in this process. William Rowe, Gerald E. Plum and Clarence Cross-man in their article alert practitioners to some of the issues that will be confronted by the lovers, families, communities and helping professionals associated with people with AIDS. Appropriate social work interventions with these groups are also outlined. In concluding this section, Carole Christensen and Tatania Kitsikis assert that social workers should take a more active role in counselling clients with genital herpes. They review the range and determinants of personal reactions found among herpes sufferers and make specific suggestions for incorporating interventive methods appropriate to aid this group of clients.

The final section of this issue is devoted to the education and teaching of professionals and the general public about STD. Steven P. Schinke, Robert F. Schilling, Marian S. Krauskopf, Gilbert J. Botvin and Mario A. Orlando describe curricula for training social workers to effectively and ethically serve persons with or at risk for AIDS and ARC. They also provide an evaluation scheme for documenting the outcomes and impacts of professional training for social work practice around AIDS issues. John R. Moore follows with a discussion of teaching methods which can be used in school or community settings to present information about the psychosocial impact of STDs. Michael Shernoff and Luis Palacios-Jimenez end this section by outlining an AIDS prevention education program primarily designed for gay and bisexual men. Concepts regarding education of the general public as well as specific suggestions for conducting effective prevention programs are provided.

This edition is concluded by an epilogue written by Allan Brandt. We hope that in reviewing these materials, readers will have been stimulated, challenged and assisted in their present and future work with the rapidly growing numbers of those who are afflicted with STD.

REFERENCES

Alberta Social Services and Community Health, Community Health Division (1985). Sexually transmitted disease – Statistical report. p. 17.
Carlton, T. & Mayes, S. (1982). Gonorrhea: Not a second class disease. *Health and Social Work,* 7(4), 301-313.

Drob, S. & Bernard, H.S. (1986). Time-limited group treatment of genital herpes patients. *International Journal Group Psychotherapy, 36*(1), 133-144.

Goudsblom, J. (1986). Public health and the civilizing process. *Milbank Quarterly, 64*(2), 161-188.

Health and Welfare Canada (1985). Sexually transmitted diseases in Canada. p. 2.

U.S. Department of Health and Human Services, Public Health Services, Centers for Disease Control (March 1986). Annual summary morbidity and mortality weekly report. *33*(54), 120.

World Health Organization (May 1987). Weekly epidemiological report. No. 19.

PART I: SOCIAL, PSYCHOLOGICAL AND MEDICAL DIMENSIONS

Sexually Transmitted Diseases — An Overview

Barbara Romanowski
Gillian Piper

INTRODUCTION

During the last five years sexually transmitted diseases (STD) have been the focus of many sensational articles in the popular press. The appearance of acquired immunodeficiency syndrome (AIDS) in 1981 and the increasing incidence of other STD worldwide has stimulated further interest in both the general public and the helping professions. The term STD has replaced the traditional "venereal diseases" (VD) which historically have included gonorrhea, syphilis, chancroid, lymphogranuloma venereum and granuloma inguinale. STD are diseases for which sexual contact is epidemiologically significant, but need not be the only mode of acquisition. Table 1 provides a list of STD. In 1984, traditional venereal diseases accounted for greater than 50% of all notifiable diseases in Canada. Although the incidence of gonorrhea has declined over the past decade, non-gonococcalurethritis (NGU) in

© 1988 by The Haworth Press, Inc. All rights reserved.

7

Table 1

Etiological Classification of

Sexually Transmitted Diseases

Bacterial

Non-gonococcal urethritis/mucopurulent cervicitis

Gonorrhea

Pelvic Inflammatory Disease

Bacterial vaginosis

Syphilis

Chancroid

Granuloma inguinale

Lymphogranuloma venereum

Viral

Herpes genitalis

Genital warts

Molluscum contagiosum

Hepatitis B

Acquired Immunodeficiency Syndrome

Cytomegalovirus Infections

Fungal

Vulvovaginitis (Candida albicans)

Protozoal

Vaginitis (Trichomonas vaginalis)

Ectoparasites

Pediculosis pubis (crab louse)

Scabies

men and mucopurulent cervicitis (MPC) in women has increased in equal proportions and now outnumbers gonorrhea by a ratio of at least 1.5:1. Furthermore the morbidity and mortality associated with NGU/MPC equals or exceeds that of gonorrhea.

Factors associated with the increasing incidence of STD include the availability of multiple sexual partners, asymptomatic disease, a highly mobile society, increasing affluence and leisure time, alcohol consumption, and variable standards in diagnosis and management. The sequelae of these infections are particularly important as they relate to maternal and infant morbidity, reproduction and fertility. For example, pelvic inflammatory disease (PID) following either mucopurulent cervicitic or gonorrhea can lead to infertility, fetal loss or infant death. Exposure to human papilloma virus (genital warts) or herpes simplex infection has been linked to the development of cancer of the cervix in women.

STD may affect any individual regardless of sex, race or socioeconomic status. Pre-pubertal children with a sexually transmitted disease should be assumed to have been sexually abused until proven otherwise.

The psychological impact of infection with an STD is often overshadowed by the medical condition. Many individuals delay attending a clinic or physician's office for diagnosis and treatment because of fear, embarrassment or guilt. Unfortunately many health care providers are equally ill at ease with STD and their interaction with the patient/client may be colored by strong feelings of disapproval or frank hostility.

Suitable management of sexually transmitted infections is dependent on the information obtained in the medical history. An individual's sexual preference and practices must be discerned as well as a history of homosexual, bisexual or heterosexual contact. This information should be acquired in a straightforward, non-judgemental fashion.

The remainder of this article deals with the most common sexually transmitted diseases. It is an attempt to supply some necessary medical information in order that appropriate sociological and psychological guidance and support can be provided to the client/patient with an STD.

NON-GONOCOCCAL URETHRITIS/MUCOPURULENT CERVICITIS (NGU/MPC)

NGU/MPC is the most common sexually transmitted disease in North America. Although the signs and symptoms of this infection are similar to that of gonorrhea the organism causing the infection is not gonorrhea and hence the term "non-gonococcal." *Chlamydia trachomatis* will be the cause of the infection in 40% to 60% of cases of NGU/MPC (Bell & Gripton, 1986). The etiology of the remaining cases is, as yet, not well defined.

The incubation period (the time between infection and the appearance of symptoms) for NGU/MPC is usually 7 to 35 days with the average being 14 to 21 days after sexual contact with an infected partner. A significant proportion of men and an extremely large proportion of women may have this infection but remain asymptomatic. These individuals can still spread the infection to their sexual partners.

The symptoms of NGU in the male are most commonly urethritis (urethral discharge) and dysuria (pain on voiding). The urethral discharge is usually less profuse and less purulent than that experienced with gonorrhea. These symptoms are sometimes only evident in the morning and the discharge can be so slight that the only recognized sign is crusting at the opening to the urinary tract.

The disease in women analogous to NGU is called mucopurulent cervicitis because the infecting organisms cause irritation of the cervix resulting in redness, swelling and an abnormal discharge (Brunham et al., 1984). Chlamydia can also infect the rectum and throat in both males and females.

Many women do not manifest any symptoms of mucopurulent cervicitis which often delays its diagnosis and treatment. The longer the infection remains untreated, the greater the chances are of progression to complications such as pelvic inflammatory disease. Locating and treating sexual partners of these women is an extremely important facet to the control and appropriate medical management of STD.

Non-gonococcal urethritis is diagnosed on the basis of a simple laboratory test which can be performed in a doctor's office. A sample of the urethral discharge is examined under the microscope to look for evidence of pus cells. In order to identify the organism causing the infection a further specimen of the discharge may be sent to the laboratory for culture. Similarly, MPC is diagnosed by examining the cervix for visual evidence of infection and then submitting a sample of the discharge for culture. However a culture is not mandatory in order to make a diagnosis of NGU.

Complications can occur if an individual is not treated promptly. In the male these complications include epididymitis (inflammation of the ducts which provide storage, transportation and maturation of sperm), prostatitis, and Reiter's syndrome which is a tetrad consisting of arthritis, urethritis, dermatitis and conjunctivitis. Females may develop acute salpingitis (inflammation of the fallopian tubes) leading to permanent tubal damage, ectopic (tubal) pregnancy, chronic pelvic pain, dysmenorrhea (painful menstruation), dyspareunia (painful sexual intercourse) and psychological morbidity. One woman in five, age 25 to 34, will become infertile after one confirmed case of salpingitis. After two to three episodes of salpingitis, 31% to 60% respectively, will become infertile (Westrom, 1980).

The final complications which must be addressed occur in infants born to infected mothers. These infants are at high risk of developing both conjunctivitis and a distinctive chlamydial pneumonia. Installation of erythromycin or tetracycline eye drops at the time of delivery will, in most cases, prevent conjunctivitis but will have no effect on the development of pneumonia. It is extremely important to check for chlamydia in pregnant women at high risk of acquiring this infection.

Non-gonococcal urethritis/mucopurulent cervicitis is a relatively easy infection to treat with antibiotics. The dosage and duration of therapy is somewhat variable depending on the specific drug utilized. It is of course important for the patient not only to take the medications properly but also to abstain from sexual contact until a test of cure has been carried out and finally to ensure treatment of his or her sexual partners.

GONORRHEA

Gonorrhea is an infection caused by the bacteria *Neisseria gonorrhoeae*. The disease is almost always sexually transmitted.

The groups at highest risk of gonorrhea are males age 20 to 24 years followed by females age 15 to 19 years. Males 15 to 19 years and females 20 to 24 years follow sequentially.

The clinical picture of the disease is varied with many individuals being asymptomatic. Only 20% to 50% of women with a genital infection will have symptoms (Hook & Holmes, 1985). The symptoms may be as slight as a change in the normal vaginal discharge but may also include dysuria, bleeding between menstrual periods or pain and swelling of the glands situated at the vaginal opening. Symptoms generally appear two to ten days after contact with an infected partner.

The most common complication of genital gonorrhea in women is pelvic inflammatory disease. The bacteria ascends from the cervix into the uterus and from there spreads to the fallopian tubes and ovaries. The sequelae of PID is often sterility or ectopic pregnancy due to scarring of the fallopian tubes thereby interfering with passage of the ova to the uterus.

Anorectal gonococcal infections in women are not uncommon and are in most instances, due to contiguous spread of infection from the vagina rather than occurring as a result of penile-anal intercourse. This type of infection is most frequently asymptomatic.

Orogenital contact can also transmit the infection. It is acquired more effectively by fellatio than cunnilingus, therefore proportionally more women and gay men will contract a pharyngeal infection. Again the majority of these infections are asymptomatic.

The vast majority of men who acquire gonococcal infections have symptoms with only 3% to 10% remaining asymptomatic. Presenting symptoms include an abrupt onset of dysuria and purulent urethral discharge.

The most common complication of untreated gonorrhea in men is acute epididymitis with pain and swelling of the testes. Damage to the epididymis can result in sterility. Other complications include infection of the prostate gland and the lymph nodes surrounding the penis.

The diagnosis of gonorrhea is made on the basis of laboratory tests in the same way as previously described for NGU/MPC. Early treatment with antibiotics is effective at both eradicating the disease and preventing complications from occurring. Once again it is extremely important that sexual partners be identified and offered appropriate treatment.

GONORRHEA IN CHILDREN

Genital gonorrhea in children should be considered the result of sexual abuse until there is definitive proof to the contrary. Research has consistently demonstrated the very infrequent transmission by means other than some type of sexual contact (Neinstein et al., 1984). Neonates born to mothers with untreated gonorrhea may develop conjunctivitis which is associated with serious complications if not recognized and treated early. Again the instillation of antibiotic eye drops at the time of delivery usually prevents this complication from occurring.

VAGINITIS

Vaginal infections are common in adult women. The three organisms most frequently found are *Candida albicans, Trichomonas vaginalis,* and *Gardnerella vaginalis* (Bowie, 1983). Infections of the vagina cause inflammation, abnormal vaginal discharge and genital itching.

Candidiasis or yeast infection is caused by a fungus — usually *Candida albicans.* Females rarely acquire this infection through sexual contact. However, women may transmit the infection to their partners resulting in an inflammation of the glans penis. Factors making women more susceptible to this infection include pregnancy, antibiotic therapy, oral contraceptive use, menstruation, diabetes mellitus and immunosuppression. Nylon underwear and pantyhose may also be contributing factors as they increase the temperature and humidity of the perineum. Following clinical/laboratory investigation to determine the causative organism, candidiasis is treated with vaginal application of antifungal creams. Unfortunately, there is a tendency for the infection to recur following treatment.

Trichomonas vaginalis (a parasite) is acquired during sexual contact with an infected individual while *Gardnerella vaginalis* (a bacteria) is rarely sexually transmitted. Both infections are manifest by an abnormal vaginal discharge, inflammation and irritation of the genital area. The discharge associated with gardnerella, tends to be slight in amount and malodorous, while that of trichomonas is profuse, purulent and frothy.

Diagnosis is made through clinical and laboratory examination. Treatment with vaginal creams and/or oral medication is usually effective. The regular male partner of an infected woman is often treated to prevent re-infection of the female partner.

GENITAL HERPES

The most common cause of genital sores in North America is infection by the *Herpes Simplex* virus (HSV). This virus is responsible not only for genital lesions but also for cold sores around the mouth. HSV is divided into two types, HSV I most often isolated from lesions around the mouth and HSV II isolated from the genital area (Corey et al., 1983). However, both types can and do infect all anatomical sites.

Transmission of the virus is by direct contact with an infected area of the body. The transmission most frequently occurs during sexual intercourse. However, it can occur during orogenital contact and can be transferred from one area of the body to another by self-inoculation. The incubation period of the virus is between two and twenty days. It is possible for the virus to be acquired, immediately become dormant and not produce a clinical episode of herpes for many months.

An outbreak of genital herpes is usually preceded by a brief period of discomfort consisting of numbness, irritation or tingling at the site of infection. This is followed by the appearance of blisters which rupture forming painful sores that heal without scar formation. The entire process occurs over a period of approximately twenty days for the initial outbreak and ten days for recurrences.

The number and severity of recurrences which occur cannot be predicted and is different for each individual. However recurrences tend to become less frequent and severe with time.

Individuals with genital herpes may transmit their infection from the time of the initial discomfort until blisters have healed completely. A very small proportion of infected individuals may continue to shed the virus although lesions are not present. For these individuals it is extremely difficult to determine when unprotected sexual intercourse is safe (Guinan et al., 1981).

The diagnosis of genital herpes is made on the basis of a clinical examination and a positive viral culture. Blood tests for the measurement of herpes antibodies are not at all useful in confirming this diagnosis (Corey & Holmes, 1983). Treatment, currently available in the form of oral acyclovir, offers the patient some control over the number and severity of their recurrences (Douglas et al., 1984). However this drug is not a cure.

There are two major problems associated with genital HSV infections, both affecting women. An association between the development of cancer of the cervix and genital herpes has been observed. It is extremely important for women with genital herpes to have Papanicolaou (PAP) smears done at least once yearly and possibly twice. Early diagnosis of cancer of the cervix increases the cure rate. The second problem involves the possibility of infecting a newborn child during delivery. Close monitoring of genital herpes during the last trimester of pregnancy is required in all women with a history of genital herpes or women whose partners have a history of genital herpes. Should the virus be found near term or lesions present at the time of delivery, consideration should be given to delivering the child by caesarean section.

SYPHILIS

Syphilis is caused by a spirochete called *Treponema pallidum*. The organism is transmitted by direct contact with an infected person and like other STD does not survive away from the body. The disease progresses through three infectious stages: primary, secondary, and early latent syphilis followed by a late latent period when the disease is not considered infectious (Romanowski & Sutherland, 1983). The infectious period of the illness is when sexual partners are at risk of acquiring the infection.

The primary stage occurs nine to ninety days after sexual contact with an infected partner has occurred. A chancre (painless ulcer) develops at the site of contact. This is usually accompanied by swollen lymph glands in the groin. The lesion will heal spontaneously in two to four weeks.

The secondary stage follows the disappearance of the chancre by two to four weeks. This stage consists of a systemic illness manifested by fever, weight loss, fatigue, and a rash which characteristically includes the palms of the hands and soles of the feet. Again the symptoms may disappear spontaneously in two to six weeks.

A latent stage, with no symptoms follows and is usually divided into early and late. During the early latent phase relapses to secondary syphilis occur in a small proportion of individuals and therefore this stage is considered infectious. Two years after the initial primary chancre the disease progresses to the late latent phase.

Studies indicate that 15% to 40% of individuals with untreated syphilis will develop tertiary disease two to forty years after the initial infection. Tertiary syphilis affects the heart and central nervous system. The advent of prompt treatment with antibiotics has certainly decreased the number of cases of tertiary syphilis seen.

The diagnosis of syphilis is made on the basis of a history, clinical examination and laboratory tests. The laboratory tests consist of a microscopic examination of the primary chancre and a blood test. This very specific test can reveal past or present infection with *Treponema pallidum*.

Treatment with antibiotics is effective at any stage of the disease. However the earlier diagnosis is made and treatment given the greater the chances are for complete recovery. As with other sexually transmitted diseases, syphilis can infect the unborn child. Screening for syphilis is therefore an important aspect of prenatal care.

ACQUIRED IMMUNODEFICIENCY SYNDROME

Acquired Immunodeficiency Syndrome (AIDS) is a viral infection causing a severe depression of the immune system. This results in the development of life threatening unusual infections and/or malignancies. The virus that causes AIDS is a retrovirus called Human

Immunodeficiency Virus (HIV). This virus was previously referred to as HTLV-III or LAV (Brodes & Gallo, 1984). The virus has been isolated in multiple body fluids including blood, semen, urine, breast milk, saliva, cerebrospinal fluid, vaginal secretions and tears.

The syndrome was first recognized and reported to the Centres for Disease Control in Atlanta, Georgia in the summer of 1981 (Fauci, 1985). Since that time there has been an escalation in the number of reported cases not only in North America, but also worldwide. The United States has reported the highest number of cases at 37,386 (U.S. Department of Health and Human Services, 1987) with the worldwide figure including the United States totalling 50,291 (National AIDS Center, 1987). Over half the reported cases have already died of this disease.

Identified high risk groups for the development of AIDS include homosexual/bisexual males, recipients of blood transfusion/blood products prior to the introduction of a blood screening program, intravenous drug abusers, heterosexual partners of individuals belonging to a high risk group, and children of parents belonging to a high risk group.

For the homosexual/bisexual group, the age of highest risk is 20 to 39 years. Current research indicates the virus to be transmitted only through infected blood and semen. By far the most common mode of transmission is through sexual contact, accounting for 70% to 80% of all cases. However, the presence of HIV antibody does not always mean the person will develop AIDS. There are three well defined clinical patterns.

Asymptomatic HIV Infection: this individual has been exposed to HIV but remains healthy. However, these patients can infect others either through sexual contact or through blood.

AIDS Related Complex (ARC): this is a clinical and laboratory syndrome characterized by significantly enlarged lymph nodes at two sites other than the groin or a constellation of clinical and laboratory abnormalities. The clinical abnormalities consist of persistent night sweats, persistent diarrhea, persistent fatigue, persistent fever, and a weight loss representing greater than 10% of the individual's normal body weight.

AIDS: the development of an unusual infection and/or specified malignancies occurring in an individual infected with HIV is defined as a case of AIDS. Individuals with AIDS have usually manifested symptoms of ARC prior to developing these infections and/or malignancies.

Pneumocystis carinii pneumonia is the most common infection and carries the highest case fatality rate. Kaposi's sarcoma, a skin cancer previously seen among elderly individuals, is the most common malignancy diagnosed in individuals with AIDS. HIV can also attack the central nervous system directly causing dementia and personality changes. To date no individuals diagnosed as having AIDS have recovered and the mean survival time is approximately thirteen months from the time of diagnosis.

Until recently treatment has been directed at the individual infections and/or malignancies. At the time this article was written a drug called azidothymidine had recently been released for use in North America. Although the drug is not a cure for AIDS it is the first agent which has affected the mean survival time of these individuals. We are all extremely hopeful that this is the first of many agents which will eventually control and cure this devastating infection.

Public education is extremely important in preventing the spread of all sexually transmitted diseases including AIDS. Individuals must be informed that AIDS is a disease primarily acquired through sexual contact and that there is no risk to individuals having casual contact with high risk patients. This disease is clearly transmitted by sexual contact, receiving infected blood or blood products, sharing contaminated intravenous equipment or by being passed from an infected mother to her unborn child. AIDS is not contracted by inanimate objects or even by shaking hands or kissing an infected individual.

A truly monogamous relationship between two uninfected individuals will certainly prevent infection. Other control measures include routine use of a condom, avoiding rectal intercourse, or oral intercourse without a condom. These precautions prevent the exchange of body fluids and thereby infection.

CONCLUSION

The education of the entire adolescent and adult population on all aspects of sexually transmitted diseases, including AIDS, must become an educational reality in an attempt to control these infections. STD can be controlled not by health authorities or school boards, but by well educated responsible individuals.

We have attempted to provide a summary of the most common sexually transmitted diseases in this article. Although this has not been an exhaustive review of the entire subject it will hopefully provide counsellors in helping professions with some basic information on which to educate and counsel individuals.

REFERENCES

Bell, T.A., Grayston, J.T. (1986). Centres for disease control guidelines for prevention and control of chlamydia trachomatis infections. *Ann Intern Medicine*, 104: 524-526.

Bowie, W.R. (1983). Vaginitis and cervicitis. *Medicine North America*, 6: 506-514.

Brodes, S., Gallo, R.G. (1984). A pathogenic retrovirus (HTLV-III) linked to AIDS. *The New England Journal of Medicine*, 311: 1292-1297.

Brunham, R.C., Paavonen, J., Stevens, C.E., Kiviat, N., Kuo, C.C., Critchlow, C.W., Homes, K.K. (1984). Mucopurulent cervicitis — the ignored counterpart in women in urethritis in men. *The New England Journal of Medicine*, 311: 1-6.

Corey, L., Holmes, K.K. (1983). Genital herpes simplex virus infections: Current concepts in diagnosis, therapy and prevention. *Ann Intern Medicine*, 98: 973-983.

Corey, L., Adams, H.G., Brown, Z.A., Homes, K.K. (1983). Genital herpes simplex virus infections: Clinical manifestations, course and complications. *Ann Intern Medicine*, 98: 958-972.

Douglas, J.M., Critchlow, C., Benedetti, J., Mertz, G.J., Connor, J.D., Hintz, M.A., Fahnlander, A., Remington, M., Winter, C., Corey, L. (1984). A double-blind study of oral acyclovir for suppression of recurrences of genital herpes simples virus infection. *The New England Journal of Medicine*, 310: 1551-1556.

Fauci, A.S. (1985). The acquired immunodeficiency syndrome: An update. *Ann Intern Medicine*, 102: 800-813.

Guinan, M.E., MacCalman, J., Kern, E. R., Overall, J.C., Spruance, S.L.

(1981). The course of untreated recurrent genital herpes simplex infection in 27 women. *The New England Journal of Medicine*, 304: 759-763.

Hook, E.W., Holmes, K.K. (1984). Gonococcal infections. *Ann Intern Medicine*, 102: 229-243.

Neinstein, L.S., Goldenring, J., Carpenter, S. (1984). Nonsexual transmission of sexually transmitted diseases: An infrequent occurrence. *Pediatrics*, 74: 67-76.

National AIDS Centre. (1987). Personal Communication.

Romanowski, B., Sutherland, R. (1983). Epidemiology and control of sexually transmitted diseases. *Medicine North America*, 6: 494-498.

United States Department of Health and Human Services. Public Health Service, Centre for Disease Control. *Morbidity and mortality weekly report*. June 15, 1987.

Westrom, L. (1980). Incidence, prevalence, and trends of acute pelvic inflammatory disease and its consequences in industrial countries. *American Journal of Obstetrics and Gynecology*, 138: 880-892.

Sexually Transmitted Diseases: Psychosocial Parameters and Implications for Social Work Practice

Marianne Wright
Margaret Rodway

INTRODUCTION

Despite the discovery of penicillin and the prophesies of the 1950s that sexually transmitted diseases (STD) would be eradicated, they continue to climb to epidemic proportions. It is now becoming obvious that there are more than medical factors contributing to the dramatic spread and increase of STD. These factors are both sociological and psychological in nature and cannot be ignored if we are to treat the person and not just the disease.

In 1986, it was reported in the United States that the incidence of gonorrhea had reached 896,383 cases and the incidence of syphilis was 67,929 (U.S. Department of Health, Education and Welfare). In Canada during 1985 the most recent date for which statistics are available, there were 43,348 reported cases of STD accounting for 56% of all notifiable diseases (Health and Welfare Canada). Of these, 40,741 cases were gonorrhea and 2,007 were syphilis. In Alberta, where this study was carried out, there were 5,980 cases of notifiable sexually transmitted diseases in 1985 (Alberta Social Services and Community Health). Gonorrhea accounted for 5,690 cases and syphilis for 90 cases. In actuality, the number of STD in Canada and the United States are much higher than those reported. Many individuals do not seek medical care for economic reasons or because they fear a social stigma or because they may experience no

© 1988 by The Haworth Press, Inc. All rights reserved.

symptoms. Pariser (1972) estimates 90% and Kampmeier (1973) 70% of all women as asymptomatic. Furthermore, many physicians do not report STD to the local health authorities or follow up on contacts. Findings from a study of Rothenberg, Bross and Vernon (1980) suggest that the number of cases of gonorrhea actually seen by private physicians may be double the number reported. It has been calculated that between 60% and 80% of gonorrhea cases go unreported by physicians in Canada (Health and Welfare Canada, 1983). Despite the availability of penicillin for treatment, gonorrhea, according to De Costa (1971), "is by far and away the most common cause of infertility in both males and females."

The statistics dramatically illustrate the seriousness of STD, yet relatively little research has been carried out in either Canada or the U.S. on the sociopsychological aspects. The most comprehensive studies have been conducted in England by physicians. These studies substantiate the supposition that STD are not just a medical problem (Mayou, 1975; Morton, 1971; Wells, 1972).

A number of studies have examined the relationship between demographic and social factors and incidence of STD (Fulford et al., 1983; Judson & Maltz, 1987; Owen & Hill, 1972; Rosebury, 1971; Secondi, 1974). A few studies have focussed on the negative effects of societal attitudes and on the impact of a diagnosis of STD on individuals (Hart, 1973; Ross, 1982; Smartt & Lightner, 1971; Tuffanelli, 1975). Indeed, Carlton and Mayes (1982), in their comprehensive review of the literature on gonorrhea, concluded that "it appears that the psychological responses of its victims have received far less attention than the physical."

Those studies that have been conducted on the psychological and emotional impact of STD have concluded that often a diagnosis of an STD can result in psychological and social problems such as anxiety, depression, insomnia, loss of appetite, feelings of guilt, and few satisfactory social relationships (Elias, 1972; Giard, 1971; Hart, 1975; Kite, 1971). These studies also suggest that the stigma attached to STD is sufficiently strong to be a factor in causing such emotional responses. As well, research indicates that emotional response to STD can take a more severe form. Mayou (1975) found that 20% of STD patients could be regarded as potential psychiatric cases and Pedder and Goldberg (1976) reported an even higher prevalence. Hart (1977) asserts that STD infection is related directly to the sociopathic personality. It should be noted, however, that these studies were often conducted with patients who attended public health STD clinics and hence, the findings are not representative of the larger population with STD.

Experts increasingly express concern over the escalating incidence of STD among the young. Youths are more sexually active at an earlier age and more likely to engage in intercourse than previous generations. The use of alcohol and drugs sets an atmosphere which can be conducive to promiscuity and, consequently, to STD. A recent survey study (O'Reilly & Aral, 1985) supports the notion that teenagers are an important component of the population at risk for STD.

In terms of psychosocial factors, Ekstom (1970) and Felstein (1974) found in their studies that young people contracting STD were often immature, had personality disorders and were from poor home backgrounds. A number of other studies (Freeven & Bannatyne, 1979; Kite, 1971; Meek, Askari & Belman, 1979; Sgroi, 1979; Terrell, 1977) found that gonorrhea in the prepubertal child is not rare, noting that it can result not only from abuse but also from nonsexual as well as sexual contact with family members. In terms of adolescents Phillips and Spence (1983) found that youths' attitudes and behavior play a major role in the increase of gonococcal infection in this group.

The spiralling increases in STD cannot be attributed to any one factor. Guthe and Idsoe (1971) have identified several including unprecedented demographic and economic change, technological development, urbanization, industrialization, the emergence of permissive behavior patterns and new attitudes towards sexuality, particularly that of prostitution and homosexuality. Schofield (1973) attributes the increase in promiscuity and subsequently STD to increased mobility, drug addiction, materialism, permissiveness, mass information and more effective contraceptions. Darrow (1975) asserts that this increase is largely a product of increased sexual activity and of the rapid acceptance of a new sexual license and freedom, which has led to a partial breakdown of traditional sex norms. The emergence of AIDS and subsequent emphasis on monogamous relationships may however somewhat reverse this trend.

The research evidence available then, points to the emotional and psychological factors which may predispose some individuals to promiscuity and to the possibility of contracting STD. The literature further identifies the social and societal pressures of our modern world which impact on this increase. It may be concluded, therefore, that either psychological or sociological factors or both in combination, contribute substantially to the epidemic proportions of STD today. However, few STD clinics employ social workers and the focus continues to be on medical causes while the statistics continue an upward climb. Because of the increasing incidence of STD, social workers in health and other social agencies are working more frequently with clients who are victims of the disease. There is an important need therefore to understand its various dimensions.

In an effort to add to existing research knowledge, the present study was undertaken in a clinic where a social worker was employed and the focus was on both psychosocial and medical aspects of the diseases.

THE SETTING

The STD Clinic in which the study was undertaken, is located in downtown Edmonton, Alberta, and serves a population of over half a million. The Clinic falls under the auspices of the Alberta Occupational and Community Health and its authority is based on the Venereal Disease Prevention Act established in 1918. Its program provides for free diagnosis and treatment, contact tracing, statistical actual number of individuals who utilize the services of the clinic. Instead statistics are kept on the number of visits to the clinic. For example, in 1985, there were 326 patient visits per week. Thus, one individual could conceivably have several clinic visits during the year.

Social work services, which began in 1974, revolve around a team approach to the treatment of the STD client. The nurses, however, are responsible for the referrals to the social worker. Each waiting room has a sign explaining the social work services and the nurses also mention the service during their discussions with the client. If the client expresses an interest in the counselling service, then they are referred to the social worker. Because statistics are kept on the number of visits rather than individuals, it is impossible to estimate what percentage are referred for counselling service.

The majority of clients seen for counselling are female, in the 15 to 19 age bracket, single, unemployed and Caucasian, although Metis and treaty Indian are frequently seen. Problems identified by the patients are varied; the two most prevalent being marital and financial, along with those of addiction, prostitution, homosexuality, depression, pregnancy and housing. Social work services vary from making referrals to more intensive counselling based on the needs and desires of the patient.

THE SAMPLE

All clients who requested counselling and who had been seen within a three month period at the STD Clinic were included in the sample. The study, therefore, does not include a random sample, nor is it representative of all STD clients. With the exception of two clients, all were seen first at the Clinic and then were referred by the nursing staff for counselling service. The two clients not referred by nursing staff were referred by other clinic counselling clients. One of those two clients had previously been treated at the Clinic, while the other was examined at the Clinic following initiation of counselling as she was bisexual and was concerned about the possibility of contact with an infected individual. Both these two clients were, therefore, considered as Clinic clients.

The existence of an STD was not a criteria for clients to be included in the sample. Many individuals seek examination at the Clinic because they have reason to believe they may have an STD, or they have been listed as a contact, or they have inordinate fear of STD. In all these cases an STD may or may not be present. However, because they have sought examination, they are eligible for counselling service. As well, some of the individuals had contracted an STD in the past and were concerned about recidivism. All clients, with the exception of two, seen in this three month time period, agreed to participate in the study. In those two instances, clients were arbitrarily excluded from the study by reason of language or reading limitations. The 20 participating clients were assured that confidentiality would be protected by altering names and any identifying information. Standardized instructions given by the researcher described the purpose of the research as that of increasing understanding and knowledge of the STD client.

MEASUREMENT INSTRUMENTS

The primary research instrument utilized for exploring the psychosocial parameters of STD was the California Psychological Inventory (CPI) (Gough, 1975). The test was chosen from a variety of other psychological testing instruments because it is relatively short, easy to administer and is an inventory of personality characteristics important for social living and social interaction. This test does not measure pathology, but it has been found to have special utility in work with delinquent and asocial behavior. As many of the STD clients seem to be immersed in a subculture, it was hoped that this test would provide some information as to dominant features in these subcultures.

The test measures eighteen facets of interpersonal psychology: dominance, capacity for status, sociability, social presence, self-acceptance, sense of well-being, responsibility, socialization, self-control, tolerance, good impression, community, achievement via conformance, achievement via independence, intellectual efficiency, psychological-mindedness, flexibility and femininity. Satisfactory data on reliability and validity of the CPI has been reported in a number of studies (Gough, 1975).

PROCEDURE

The CPI was briefly explained to the 20 clients involved. The client was then placed in a private office where he/she could complete the test. Each was told to answer the questions to the best of his/her ability and if they found it impossible to answer any question, then to leave it blank. The majority of clients answered all questions. No time limit was imposed, although the estimated time for completion is forty-five minutes to one hour. Testing time varied from forty-five minutes to one and one half hours with the exception of one individual who took two hours. Each individual was given the opportunity to review the test results for their own information or learning.

In terms of demographic data, the following characteristics were explored: age, racial origin, marital status, confirmed venereal infection, education, parental material status, past and present nonmedical use of drugs, frequency of hospitalization for psychiatric care, patient identified problems and frequency of abortion.

RESULTS

The purpose of this exploratory descriptive study was to examine some of the psychosocial parameters of STD through an analysis of 20 clients who attended an STD disease clinic and requested counselling from a social worker. Through psychological testing and demographic characteristics, data were gathered for analysis of the 20 counselling clients to ascertain what could be learned about them, their background and the influence of subcultures that could have impact for a more comprehensive understanding of STD. Some of the findings were generally consistent with those cited in the literature review. More specifically, the demographic data revealed that the majority of counselling patients were single (60%) or divorced (10%), Caucasian (75%) and over 20 years of age (90%) with 45% in the 20 to 24 year age bracket. When the most recently available general population statistics for Alberta were examined, it was found that 21.3% were single; 2.5% were divorced; 7.6% were over 20 years of age with 11.8% in the 20 to 24 year age bracket (Statistics Canada, 1981).

The majority of the sample were not employed (55%) nor had they completed high school (55%). This compared with an unemployment rate of 9% for Alberta, while in terms of education, 41% of the general population have completed high school.

Over 85% of the sample had been involved in previous nonmedical use of drugs and over 80% were presently involved. Whether or not the 80% of the sample presently using drugs nonmedically are in fact dependent on drugs is difficult to estimate, particularly because 35% of the sample used marijuana only and there is considerable controversy over the addictive qualities of this drug.

Almost half (40%) of the sample had been hospitalized at least once for psychiatric reasons. It is difficult to compare hospitalization for psychiatric reasons with the general population because available statistics are based on a number of discharges. Statistics for 1982 indicate that there were 16,253,000 discharges from hospitals for individuals with mental disorders (Statistics Canada, 1981).

It was also noted that 53% of the females in the sample have had therapeutic abortions. The statistics for Alberta reveal that of women aged 15 to 44 years, 2% had abortions in 1981 (Statistics Canada, 1981).

Statistics for the Alberta population were not available for social origin or parental marital status, so comparisons could not be made on this data. In summary, based on the comparisons made, it can be stated that the sample indicated higher rates than the Alberta population on the following dimensions: single and divorced status; over 20 years of age; unemployed; completed high school; nonmedical use of drugs; psychiatric hospitalization and abortion.

When the data derived from the psychological testing were examined by factor analysis further psychosocial dimensions were identified some of which had not been cited in the previous studies cited. (See Table 1.)

More specifically, it was determined that the majority of respondents to the California Psychological Inventory presented evidence of deprivation in their childhoods, accounting for immaturity in their behavior as evidenced by impulsive behavior, with little or no self-control. They appeared to lack inner controls on their behavior or more simply, they did not feel they were in control or their own lives. Furthermore, the data suggested that they rejected external controls on their behavior.

Evidence as to their social functioning appeared more positive indicating that the majority experienced some comfort and confidence in this area. However, there were indications that their comfort level decreased rapidly when faced with new and unfamiliar situations. This could indicate comfort at their peer level with little motivation to change.

The respondents further revealed, through testing, that there was an emphasis on personal pleasure and gain accompanied by distrust of those in authority. The test also indicated that there was a disbe-

TABLE 1. Frequency and percentage of scale scores on the three CPI factors.

	Frequency							Percent	
C.P.I. FACTORS	Extremely High	Very High	High	Normal	Low	Very Low	Extremely Low	Normal	Normal or Above
Factor 1									
Self-control	0	0	0	3	7	8	2	84	15
Good impression	0	0	0	7	8	4	1	65	35
Well-being	0	0	0	3	3	4	10	85	15
Achievement via conformance	0	0	0	3	3	9	5	85	15
Factor 2									
Dominance	0	0	3	8	5	4	0	45	55
Sociability	0	0	3	6	7	3	1	55	45
Self-acceptance	0	1	2	9	8	0	0	40	60
Capacity for status	0	0	1	4	8	2	5	75	25
Social presence	0	0	1	12	5	1	1	35	65
Factor 3									
Achievement via independence	0	1	0	10	3	5	1	45	55
Flexibility	0	2	6	10	2	0	0	10	90
Tolerance	0	0	0	5	5	4	6	75	25
Intellectual efficiency	0	0	0	3	8	3	6	85	15
Psychological-mindedness	0	0	0	6	10	4	0	70	30

lief in their own intellectual capabilities. Additionally, little stress was placed on self-analysis or self-understanding. The femininity scale revealed that the four male homosexuals scored high to extremely high on this scale, whereas the three lesbians scored normal and below on femininity. Female heterosexuals scored from low to very high and the one male heterosexual scored normal.

Regarding the possible existence and characteristics of subcultures, it was necessary to draw on all the data. Case histories and demographic data revealed that the majority (60%) of the sample appeared to exist in a subculture that did not censure the nonmedical use of drugs. They gave indication of choosing a peer level in which they felt some comfort and identity. The peer level chosen and the particular subculture in which the majority of these patients revolved seemed to emphasize the use of drugs and alcohol and promiscuous behavior. Ten percent of the sample existed in a lesbian subculture while 20% existed in a gay subculture. The latter two were similar to the straight subculture to the degree that there was acceptance of the use of drugs and there was a feeling of ease and identity within their groups. Demographic data confirmed that the majority of the sample were infected with STD.

It should be noted that the California Psychological Inventory was not only a descriptive instrument for this study, but was utilized as means for the patient's own growth. With the exception of one individual, all the sample wished to review their CPI profiles. None of them were especially surprised by what the profile revealed. Instead, the profile only confirmed what they were experiencing and identified areas of special concern that could be focused on in the counselling process. As well, the patients expressed pleasure at being asked to participate in this study because of the focus on the human rather than the disease entity of STD.

CONCLUSIONS AND IMPLICATIONS

In conclusion, this study indicates that for some individuals, STD are a symptom of stress and distress in their lives. It supports the conclusions derived by other researchers and adds additional information on the psychosocial aspects of STD that have repercussions on recidivism as well as on increasing incidence. This suggests the need for a multidisciplinary response in which social work's contribution could be significant.

There are several limitations to this study which should be mentioned. First, the sample was not randomly selected. Rather, it studied a sample which was referred for and accepted counselling services and could, therefore, be seen as motivated for change. Second, the sample size was limited. Ideally it should have been much larger and examined over a longer period of time. Finally, the sample was comprised mainly of individuals from the lower socioeconomic group. It appears that many, if not most, middle and upper class individuals seek treatment from their own physicians and hence would not be part of such a study.

In the STD clinic which was the setting for the present study, all clients who expressed any concerns beyond their physical symptoms, were informed that counselling was part of the service offered. However, there was no pressure exerted by the staff for clients to seek such help. The twenty clients in the study all requested counselling on the basis of their awareness that personal problems existed for which they needed help. The problems they most frequently cited during the counselling process were: unemployment, depression, alcohol or drug abuse, difficulty with family and social relationships, anxiety and difficulty in finding housing. All clients, because they had agreed to counselling, were motivated. This would not necessarily be the case generally for clients who attended a clinic where counselling was part of the service offered. Particular interventive skills would be necessary for this latter group. It should be noted that although the study group was motivated for counselling, they were hard to reach in the sense that they felt overwhelmed by their problems. All expressed feelings of anxiety, fear and apprehension about the counselling process and feelings of degradation, cheapness, dirtiness, anger at selves, humiliation and shame regarding the confirmation that they had STD.

The social worker's approach was based on assessment of the needs of the client resulting in referrals or involvement in a counselling process, or both. In those cases where referrals for other services were indicated, the social worker would generally initiate the referrals and follow up on the outcome of the referrals. Where counselling was indicated, a verbal contract was established with the client. This contract was mutually agreed upon and outlined the duration of the counselling process and responsibilities of both the client and social worker in that process. The social worker also developed a treatment plan based on the needs of the client, a diagnostic assessment and the strengths and limitations of both the client and the social worker. Any contract and treatment plan allowed for flexibility and alteration based on the counselling process. During the counselling process the social worker continued to check her own reactions to the client.

The counselling itself involved the establishment of a trusting relationship often begun through a comprehensive history taking. The focus, however, was not on the past but on the present and future and on the realities confronting the client. The emphasis was often on their personal relationships as many clients suffered from loneliness, alienation and depression. As well, depending upon the needs of the clients, counselling included a thorough discussion of STD and their mental and emotional reaction to both the disease and its implications for their lives.

In essence, the purpose of counselling was to help the client achieve better personal and social functioning. Therefore, it was geared to the client as an individual, a family member, a member of a subculture, and a member of society.

At an STD clinic, the social worker is daily confronted with often overwhelming societal and emotional problems. To see beyond such labels as "an STD client" to the often vulnerable human being who is experiencing pain and turmoil is the most important task of the social worker. To care for that human being and to respect their dignity and unique individuality is essential, for they will not return if they are not valued as worthwhile. Responsibility entails listening, confronting, and caring about the patient's needs not just during the interview but also after they leave the office.

The requisite knowledge and skills that have been outlined for work with STD patients have appeared consistently in the social work literature over the years as generic to work with a variety of client populations. For example, Chilman (1975) and Tversky and Cale (1976) have pinpointed social work's particular emphasis on helping individuals improve their social functioning as essential in this aspect. It is, therefore, concluded that social work has a crucial role to play in a comprehensive treatment program for such clients and that social workers should be part of clinic staff. More specifically, many of the factors that need to be considered in attempts to improve treatment in STD clinics have been noted by a number of authors as variables with which social workers have expertise (Brown, 1961; Dahlke, Carlton, Itzkowitz, & Madison, 1980; Dunbar & Jackson, 1972; Felstein, 1974; Seabury, 1971; Walz, Willenbring, & de Moll, 1974).

A final implication emerging from the study suggests that a team approach to a treatment program could more effectively meet the physical and emotional needs of the clients through the combination of expertise. The social worker could offer to the STD treatment team, a number of services. First, they could provide an emotional outlet for clients thus freeing time for medical practitioners. There is often a strong emotional response to contracting sexually transmitted diseases and in some cases, the client's response can be severe requiring time away from prescribed duties by nursing staff. Second they could offer environmental support and services to the patients through referrals for alcohol/drug treatment, employment counselling, housing agencies and welfare institutions. Finally, they could provide an understanding to medical and nursing staff of the psychological and sociological implications and ramifications of STD through inservice training and staff development.

Such a team approach is not without its difficulties. First and foremost, both medical and social work professionals must work cooperatively towards the prime objectives — treating the person. If that objective becomes blurred by petty rivalries or power struggles, the client will be the one to suffer and the team concept will crumble. Thus, roles need to be clearly delineated with areas of responsibilities outlined, and staff chosen who are responsible professionals with a commitment towards the team concept as a treatment resource for the client.

REFERENCES

Alberta Social Services and Community Health, Community Health Division (1985). Statistical report, sexually transmitted disease control.

Brown, E.L. (1961). Things as familiar and comforting symbols. In *Newer dimensions of patient care*, Part 1; 30-54. New York: Russel Sage Foundation.

Carlton, T.O. & Mayes, S.M. (1982). Gonorrhea: Not a second class disease. *Health and Social Work*, 7(4), 301-13.

Chilman, C. (1975, Spring). Some knowledge bases about human sexuality for social work education. *Journal of Education for Social Work*, 8-12.

Dalke, 0., Carlton, T.O., Itzkowitz, C., & Madison, T.M. (1980). *A foundation for social policy analysis.* Lexington, Mass.: Ginn Custom Publishing, 2-6.

Darrow, W.W. (1975, March). Changes in sexual behavior and venereal diseases. *Clinical Obstetrics and Gynecology*, 11, 223-232.

De Costa, E.J. (1971). Implications of gonorrhea. In *The V.D. crisis*, New York: Pfizer, 37.

Dunbar, E. & Jackson, J. (1972, September). Free clinics for young people. *Social Work*, 17, 35-39.

Ekstom, K. (1970). Patterns of sexual behavior in relation to venereal disease. *British Journal of Venereal Disease*, 46, 93-95.

Elias, J. (1972). *The venereal disease crisis*. New York: Pfitzer.

Felstein, Ivor. (1974). *Sexual pollution: The fall and rise of venereal disease.* London: David and Charles Publishers, 115.

Freeven, T.C. & Bannatyne, R.M. (1979, August). Gonococcal vulvovaginitis in prepubertal girls. 19, 491-493.

Feelford, K.W., Catteral, R.D., Hainville, E., Lim, K.S., & Wilson, G.D. (1983). Social and psychological factors in the distribution of STD in male clinic attenders. *British Journal of Venereal Disease*, 59, 376-80.

Giard, R. (1971, October). Influence of gonococcal urethritis in men in their psychiatric state. *British Journal of Venereal Disease*, 47, 379-403.

Gough, H.C. (1975). *Manual for the California psychological inventory*. Palo Alto: Consulting Psychologists Press, 5.

Guthe, T. & Idsoe, O. (1971). In R.S. Morton, *Sexual freedom and venereal disease*. London: Peter Owen, 188.

Hart, G. (1973). Psychological aspects of venereal disease in a war environment. *Social Science and Medicine*, 7, 455-467.

Hart, G. (1975, March). Role of preventive methods in the control of venereal disease. *Clinical Obstetrics and Gynecology*, 18, 243-253.

Hart, G. (1977). *Sexual malady and disease: An introduction to modern venereology*. Chicago: Nelson-Hall.

Health and Welfare Canada, Bureau of Epidemiology. (1985). *Sexually transmitted disease in Canada*. Ottawa.

Judson, F.N. & Maltz, A.B. (1978, October-December). A rational basis for the epidemiologic treatment of gonorrhea in a clinic for sexually transmitted disease. *Sexually Transmitted Diseases*, 5, 89-92.

Kampmeier, R.H. (1973, September). Venereal disease control. *American Journal of Hospital Pharmacology*, 30, 774-780.

Kite, E. (1971, April). Good personality breakdown in venereology. *British Journal of Venereal Disease*, 47, 136-145.

Mayou, R. (1975, February). Psychological morbidity in a clinic for sexually transmitted disease. *British Journal of Venereal Disease*, 51(1), 57-60.

Meek, L.M., Askari, A., & Belman. (1979, October). Prepubertal gonorrhea. *Journal of Urology*, 122, 534.

Morton, R.S. (1971). *Sexual freedom and venereal disease*. London: Peter Owen.

O'Reilly, K.R. & Aral, S.O. (1985). Adolescence and sexual behavior: Trends and implications for STD. *Journal of Adolescent Health Care*, 6(4), 262-270.

Owen, R.L. & Hill, J.R. (1972, June 5). Rectal and pharyngeal gonorrhea in homosexual men. *Journal of the American Medical Association*, 220, 1311-1323.

Pariser, H. (1972, September). Asymptomatic gonorrhea. *Medical Clinics of North America*, 65(5), 1127-1132.

Pedder, J.R. & Golberg, V.P. (1976). A survey by questionnaire of psychiatric disturbance in patients attending a V.D. clinic. *British Journal of Venereal Disease*, 46, 58-61.

Phillips, S. & Spence, M.R. (1983). Medical and psychosocial aspects of gonococcal infection in the adolescent patient: Epidemiology, diagnosis and treatment. *Journal of Adolescent Health Care*, 4(2), 138-134.

Rosebury, T. (1971). *Microbes and Morals*. New York: Viking Press, 232-265.

Ross, M.W. (1982). Social factors in homosexually acquired venereal disease. *British Journal of Venereal Disease*, 58, 263-268.

Rothenberg, R., Bross, D.C., & Vernon, T.M. (1980, September). On reports and rapport in V.C. control. *American Journal of Public Health*, 70, 946-947.

Schofield, M. (1973, October). V.D. and the young. *New Society*, 135-137.

Seabury, B.A. (1971, October). Arrangement of physical space in social work settings. *Social Work*, 16, 43-49.

Secondi, J.J. (1974). *For people who make love*. New York: Taplinger Publishing Co. 8.

Sgroi, S.M. (1979, May). Pediatric gonorrhea beyond infancy. *Pediatrics Annuls*, 8, 327-339.

Smartt, W. & Lightner, A.G. (1971, January). The gonorrhea epidemic and its control. *Medical Aspects of Human Sexuality*, 5, 97-108.

Statistics Canada, 1981 Census of Canada.

Terrell, M.E. (1977, November). Identifying the sexually abused child in a medical setting. *Health and Social Work*, 2, 121-136.

Tiversky, R.K. & Cale, W.M. (1976, Fall). Social work fees in medical care: A review of the literature and report of a survey. *Social Work in Health Care*, 2, 77.

Tuffanelli, D.F. (1975, February). Office procedures for diagnosing and testing suspected V.D. *Medical Aspects of Human Sexuality*, 9, 53-65.

U.S. Department of Health and Human Services, Public Health Services, Centre for Disease Control. (1987). *Morbidity, mortality weekly report*. 35(53), 811-813.

Walz, T., Willenbring, G., & de Moll, L. (1974, January). Environmental design. *Social Work*, 19, 38-46.

Wells, P.W.P. (1972, September). A personality study of V.D. patients using the psychoticism, extroversion, neuroticism inventory. *British Journal of Venereal Disease*, 56(5), 1101-1104.

Acquired Immunodeficiency Syndrome and Minorities: Policy Perspectives

Leon Williams
June Hopps

INTRODUCTION AND BACKGROUND

Acquired Immune Deficiency Syndrome (AIDS) has taken on the dimensions of an epidemic and has forced America to come to grips with some grim realities. There are currently 37,386 persons with AIDS, either actively ill or carriers of the disease (U.S. Department of Health and Human Services, 1987). Of these, best estimates are that 100 percent are expected to die of the illness (Boston Globe, 1986). As the epidemic increases in magnitude and strength, it is projected that by the year 1991, 270,000 people will have contracted the disease and barring a medical breakthrough, will die. According to Dr. James Curran (1986), head of the federal government's Centres for Disease Control's task force on AIDS, 244,000 new cases will be diagnosed in the next five years and in 1991, 174,000 AIDS patients will be hospitalized. Their hospital costs alone will be 8 billion dollars, depending on whether a bill of 46,000 or 92,000 dollars per patient is a correct estimate (Curran, quoted in Boston Globe, 10-6-86, p. 14). Initially, there was thought to have been a limited incubation period associated with the disease of about three to five years, but recent evidence has proven that assumption to be false, suggesting that the period might be far longer—up to ten years in some instances. About 82 percent or AIDS patients develop one or both of two rare opportunistic illnesses: pneumocystis carnii pneumonia (PCP), which is a parasitic

© 1988 by The Haworth Press, Inc. All rights reserved.

infection of the lungs, and a type of cancer known as Kaposi's sarcoma (KS) which appears as blue-purple or brownish spots on the body (Dowdle, 1986).

Hundreds of thousands of dollars are being invested in research and in the treatment of AIDS victims but the prognosis remains grim, despite the advent of several new drugs among which are AZT (azidothymidine) which eases the symptoms of the disease with varying effects (Foreman, 1986). Few issues in history have enjoined more sectors of the population than this disease . . . business leaders fear that the disease may bankrupt the insurance industry, while the medical experts fear the same fate for the health care industry. Medicaid administrators brace themselves for the debate over scarce resources being allocated for the expensive care of a relatively small number of recipients and even voice concern that, when a "cure" is found, the cost to treat or prolong life may carry too high a price tag (O'Hara & Stangler, 1986). Ninety-five percent of the AIDS cases reported to date have occurred among the following groups:

—Homosexual and bisexual men, 73 percent;
—Present or past users of intravenous (IV) drugs, 17 percent (in addition, 11 percent of homosexual and bisexual men report having used IV drugs);
—Persons who have had transfusions with blood or blood products, 2 percent;
—Persons with hemophilia or other blood clotting disorders, 1 percent;
—Persons with heterosexual contacts with persons who have AIDS or are at risk of AIDS, 1 percent; and
—Infants born to infected mothers, 1 percent. (Dowdle, 1986)

AIDS cases have been reported in all fifty states, the District of Columbia, and three United States territories. Ninety percent of those cases have occurred among persons twenty through forty-nine years old, and all races have been affected. No patient is known to have recovered lost immune system function. More than 11,000 AIDS patients (54 percent) have died including 71 percent of those whose illness was diagnosed before July 1984. These statistics do not show the whole picture. Epidemiological studies suggest that as many as one million Americans may be infected by the virus that causes AIDS. Many of those persons show no signs of infection and do not know they carry the virus. Even if they show no symptoms, they may be capable of transmitting the virus for the rest of their lives (Dowdle, p. 15).

The problem with AIDS exists not so much in relation to its most visible victims, those persons or groups who have won public sympathy and now enjoy media attention, but the invisible victims, the persons who have little or no voice and who fail to conform to the profile of the typical AIDS victim. These victims have little clout and little visibility, and have become victims on the lowest reaches of a hierarchy of victims. Admittedly, all AIDS sufferers are identified with groups scorned by society but some are more scorned than others . . . prostitutes, drug addicts, marginal persons generally unconnected to family or kin, and with the least access to formal, traditional social services. A large proportion of these persons are persons of colour. As the cost of caring for the AIDS patients mount, it is this group which will be most likely overlooked in an atmosphere calling for the rationing of scarce resources.

Social work and the social services are only beginning to come to grips with the enormous consequences of AIDS for individuals and families and the problems the disease may visit upon the practice of social work. Given the profession's decade (or more) retreat from those service sectors in which contact with AIDS victims is most likely (Dieppa, 1984), the outlook for a rational and focussed response from social work is less than optimistic. This article will attempt to make the case for an appropriate social work response, and illuminate some of the issues created by AIDS for minorities in order to broaden the scope of the debate relative to the policy and service delivery problems created by the epidemic.

THE NATURAL HISTORY OF AIDS

AIDS was isolated in 1984 from human blood. Named HTLV-III, human T-lymphotropic virus type III, currently referred to as HIV-I, the virus selectively attacks a specific group of white blood cells crucial to the body's immune system. The virus also was discovered to have an affinity for infecting cells of the brain. Structurally and biochemically the AIDS virus belongs to a family of viruses called retroviruses found not only in humans but in animals, from reptiles to primates. Retroviruses do not always cause disease in their hosts. They are not living organisms, lacking the machinery and energy-generating properties to reproduce, they must exploit the cells of living organisms to perform those functions for them as the cells reproduce so does the virus (Gonda, 1986).

AIDS was presumably introduced into the United States in the 1970s but was not recognized clinically until 1981. Although no one knows whether the HIV induced syndrome is a new disease or where it came from, serologic data are now accumulating which suggests the disease was in Africa at least a decade before it came to the U.S., probably via Haiti (Gonda, p. 80). This is deduced primarily from laboratory data. Scientists have found an animal virus which may have given rise to a human variant such as AIDS. STV-III (simian T-lymphotropic virus type III) causes an AIDS-like syndrome in the macaque monkey. Moreover, antibodies to the AIDS virus exits in the blood of otherwise healthy African green monkeys. There is at least the possibility of a monkey retrovirus giving rise to the human variant of AIDS (Gonda, p. 81).

It is suspected that the AIDS virus existed in humans in central Africa for hundreds of thousands of years, but that it resided in an isolated population. Such isolated groups may have coadapted with the virus, lessening the severity of the disease and allowing for mutual coexistence. The persistence of AIDS may have been assisted by old customs such as scarification and the shared use of sharp instruments (needles) in body marking. Ethnographically, the past 30 years have seen Africa's family and geographical boundaries broken down as urbanization has intensified. Such changes have brought a virulent infectious agent into contact with previously unexposed populations, both local and international, and with devastating consequences (Gonda, p. 81). One has only to witness the effects of the tuberculosis baccilus, introduced by Europeans, on our native American population for an historical example of such exposure.

The World Health Organization (W.H.O.) reports that a minimum of 10,000 cases annually may be occurring in Africa (Knox,

1986a). They also recorded 50,291 cases of AIDS world-wide, 74 percent of which are in America (National AIDS Centre, 1987). Twenty-two European countries have reported sharp increases; from 1,630 cases as of the beginning of the year to 3,127 in July 1986 (Netter, 1986). According to Mahler (1986) AIDS is a heterosexual disease in Africa. It is spread by ordinary sexual contact between men and women, from pregnant women to their unborn children and through breast feeding (quoted in McLaughlin, 1986). In the U.S. the fact of heterosexual transmission has placed a chilling new perspective on AIDS, has broadened the scope of the problem, and generated greater public alarm.

There are three major groups of infected persons:

1. There are those with "active" or "frank" AIDS (5-10%);
2. Those with AIDS-related conditions or "complex" (ARC) (25-30%); and
3. Those who are asymptomatic for AIDS (55-60%). (U.S. Department of Health and Human Services, 1986; Grieco, 1986)

The latter two categories do not usually face imminent death. They do have significant problems caused by their ambiguous disease status and the need to make major changes in their behaviour. These persons are not only more likely to engage in sex or IV drug use than are the physically debilitated people with AIDS, but are probably more infectious as well (U.S. Department of Health and Human Services, p. 10). The treatment of choice for the latter groups has been education designed to change established sexual practices or habits of drug use. They must be warned that they are presumed at risk and infectious to others and will remain so for life.

THE PROBLEM OF AIDS
FOR PERSONS OF COLOUR

Aside from the obvious medical complications, the major impact of AIDS has been the fear foisted on the society by the nature of the disease. On the surface, it would appear that AIDS is a straightfor-

ward public health problem which would call forth the normal public health responses – isolation, inoculation and in extreme cases,
quarantine.

The disease has not responded to any known public health
method. There is no likelihood of a cure or a vaccine any time in the
future. Many observers have remarked, however, on the widespread public fear of contagion and the "wait and see" attitude
of public officials which has greeted the epidemic (O'Hara &
Stangler, p. 8). Aside from epidemiologists and a core of dedicated
medical professionals, ambivalence is the best way to characterize
the current public attitude toward AIDS. The federal government,
for example, under the influence of the Gramm-Rudman budget
reductions, has confined its role strictly to one of finding a cure for
AIDS primarily through the Centre for Disease Control (CDC) in
Atlanta, Georgia. (Note: the U.S. Congress passed landmark legislation in 1985 [P.L. 99-177] that was aimed at reducing the Federal
deficit to zero by FY 1991. The legislation was sponsored by Sena-
tors Phil Gramm [R-Tex], Warren Rudmann [R-NH], and Ernest
Hollins [D-SC] and has come to be known as the Gramm-Rudman
Bill [Washington Social Legislation Bulletin, January 1986].)
Thus, the enormous costs of caring for AIDS patients and of controlling the disease has been relegated to state and local governments (O'Hara & Stangler, p. 12). It is the authors' view that the
disconcerting association of AIDS with certain stigmatized groups,
particularly homosexuals and persons of colour, accounts for a considerable amount of the ambivalence. In the haste to find answers,
epidemiologists have inadvertently produced scapegoats for public
fear in the persons of homosexuals and inevitably, blacks (through
the African-Haitian link). As many in the gay community have observed, the country seems to have accommodated to the idea that
AIDS is a homosexual problem and are willing to see the disease
run its course out of antigay sentiments (see Morin & Batchelor,
1984). Acknowledging the African connection to AIDS puts black
Americans in a similar position.

To date, the major focus of attention in the AIDS epidemic has
been the gay community as the population at risk. This has both
positive and negative aspects. On the positive side, the attention
given to the plight of gay victims has produced beneficial results

through the dramatic presentation of individual life histories in the media. Our knowledge of the disease and awareness of its ravages have come largely through the efforts of members of the gay community who have willingly sacrificed their privacy and self esteem in order to educate the public. This has resulted in increased public support for combatting the disease and a level of awareness which has lessened the hysteria. It has not, however, enabled the public to focus on the fundamental fact of AIDS as a universal problem, heterosexual in scope and except in Africa, a disease of urban life in all its complexities. The major outbreaks are in our major cities . . . San Francisco, Los Angeles, New York, and Chicago. These are our major population centres housing a sizeable proportion of persons of colour. In New York, it is reported that 24 percent of the AIDS victims are black or hispanic quite out of proportion to their population share (Ivey, 1985).

On the other hand, the AIDS question has come to be dominated by and associated in the public perception with gays, and thus, tends to be too narrowly focussed on a category of people. As Desjarias (1986) an epidemiologist in the New York State Health Department observes, "the bottom line is that AIDS is spread by behaviour, not labels" (quoted in Miller, 1986). In this instance, a group of people have come to represent a disease and have become the focus of attention for a problem having far broader implications for public health and safety. The behaviour in question is behaviour that facilitates the transmission of the AIDS virus from one human host to another, mainly through the exchange of bodily fluids; blood, semen, saliva. Gays are not the only persons who are statistically capable of this behaviour, they are simply the primary victims at this stage in the natural history of the disease. Forecasts suggest the disease is growing more prevalent and will claim a wider range of victims, both homosexual and heterosexual (Knox, 1986b).

The gay community's response to the AIDS epidemic has been understandably defensive as the disease is associated with issues of sexual preference, human rights and individual freedom. Questions raised in this context about the consequences of gay sexual behaviour are often viewed in the gay community as attacks against gay lifestyle and values (Luehrs, Orlebeke, & Merlis, 1986). In theory, this defensive militancy has created a type of AIDS-pariah group of typically affluent white males, highly visible, urbane and articulate, who are in direct contrast to the average victim who is black or a person of colour. The general tendency in the current debate is to focus more attention on gay lifestyle and the issue of sexual preference and this has biased the social response to the AIDS epidemic. Martha Moran (1986), coordinator of a Boston conference on Women and AIDS, amplifies this concern by noting that up until now, we have perceived AIDS as a gay, white male disease. Conference leaders noted, among other things, that women account for 7 percent of those in the United States who have contracted AIDS . . . and more than half are Black and Hispanic. Many have children, some of whom also have AIDS or AIDS related conditions (ARC). Conference leaders estimate that up to 70 percent of AIDS cases in Boston might be people of colour (Bickelhaupt, 1986). In actuality, all victims of AIDS are tarred with a common brush—the gay agenda which is designed to forestall a homophobic public backlash. It follows that the needs of other victims are less ardently defended.

THE AIDS PANIC

There is a "finger in the dike" attitude in most of the pronouncements about AIDS. Health professionals and others have gone to great lengths to assure the public that there is no great cause for alarm. As the mass of negative data mounts so do the efforts of public spokespersons who would calm our fears. A public that reads articles depicting AIDS as a modern version of the bubonic plague will not be easily assuaged. It is important to remember, most parents of school aged children do not want a course in epidemiology. They simply want a guarantee that their children will not be infected. Unfortunately science does not give too many guarantees regarding AIDS—other than the disease is spreading (Dowdle, p. 17). What concerns the authors is the residue of hostility toward those groups harbouring the disease seems to be flourishing. The backlash that many gays feared seems to be making a belated appearance. There has been a little documented increase in violence directed at gays and AIDS victims talk of being shunned, not out of fear of contagion, but due to the outright hostility of co-workers and acquaintances. State and federal statutes seem to have become more punitive and less permissive. This potential for hostility is even greater if public awareness mounts regarding the AIDS-Africa link.

Combined with antigay sentiments, the resulting atmosphere of homophobic-racism may have destructive possibilities with regard to a sane and rational solution to the AIDS problem. Confinement, isolation, and a suspension of human rights are all potential results of a growing public outrage and the targets are most likely to be the traditional victims of oppression, the poor, the defenseless, and persons of colour who are inordinately present among those groups.

A 1986 U.S. Justice Department ruling involving AIDS in the workplace is an example of a growing repressive trend. It was ruled that some employers may legally fire AIDS victims if their motive is to protect other workers. This ruling resolved a debate within the government as to whether AIDS victims are handicapped persons protected by the Rehabilitation Act of 1973 which prohibits discrimination against the handicapped in federal agencies and in organizations that receive federal funds. In his opinion, Assistant Attorney General Charles J. Cooper (1986) wrote that discrimination based on physical disability caused by AIDS might be a violation of the law, but, he added, the statute does not restrict measures taken to prevent the spread of disease. The result is that an AIDS victim whose abilities are impaired may have protection against dismissal, but a fully functioning AIDS carrier may not . . . as long as dismissal is based on fear of contagion (quoted in Clark, McDaniel et al., 1986).

Since this article was initially drafted, the U.S. Supreme Court has ruled, in the case of the Nassau County (Florida) School Board v. Gene Arline, that victims of some contagious diseases are covered by the same laws that protect handicapped workers from on-the-job bias; especially Section 504 of the Rehabilitation Act of 1973 that prevents discrimination against "otherwise qualified" handicapped persons (Press & McDaniel, 1987). Nonetheless, a variety of new laws are being proposed and enacted in several states which signal a more conservative backlash. In California, for example, a new initiative sponsored by backers of the now out-of-favor political extremist Lyndon Larouche, was certified to be put on the ballot in the November 1986 elections. This initiative would give broad powers to state officials to contain AIDS, including quarantine. Alabama has proposed legislation which would require AIDS testing for marriage with the results appended to the license, would quarantine inmates with AIDS and would require doctors who treat or examine suspected AIDS patients to report them to the department of health. Florida would separate children with AIDS from the school population, dismiss teachers with AIDS and require tests if there was probable cause. West Virginia would define intentional transmission of AIDS as first or second degree murder (O'Hara & Stangler, p. 12). This is only a sample of new initiatives being proposed nationwide which show a disturbing tendency toward greater punitiveness towards AIDS victims, corresponding to the pattern of conservative and fundamentalistic representation in various states and locales. The visceral response of the noninfected is to confine and punish gays and intravenous drug users (Freeman, 1986).

BEHAVIOURAL AND PSYCHOSOCIAL FACTORS IN MINORITY VICTIMS OF AIDS

Infection with the AIDS virus causes extreme physical, emotional and psychological stress for most people diagnosed with AIDS. Anxiety and depression are the most common symptoms, according to The U.S. Department of Health and Human Services (1986). Distress is evident in the preoccupation with illness and imminent death characteristic of many patients with cancer and other often fatal illnesses. The stress response at the time of diagnosis may be marked by disbelief, numbness, and inability to face the facts of the illness. Patients become angry at the illness; at the discrimination which often accompanies it; at the prospect of a lonely painful death; at the lack of effective treatment; and at medical staff, and themselves. Those who see themselves as innocent or involuntary victims of the virus having contracted it, for example, from blood transfusions, or through sexual contact with a bisexual partner, are especially prone to anger (U.S. Department of Health & Social Services, 1986).

Guilt develops, in many cases, about the disease, about past behaviour and styles of living, or about the possibility of having transmitted it to others. Sadness, hopelessness, helplessness, withdrawal, isolation and other symptoms of acute depression are present. Many patients contemplate suicide, some actually try, but few actually kill themselves. Because both physical and social support are needed, a strong network of friends and family is especially important. But homosexual and intravenous drug users who are estranged from family may lack such support, owing to rejection and/ or having few natural supports as a matter of course. Anxiety may take the form of tension, tachycardia, agitation, insomnia, anorexia and panic attacks (U.S. Department of Health & Human Services, 1978; Batchelor & Morin, 1984).

As a general rule, the most prevalent ego defense employed by AIDS victims is that of denial . . . an inability to accept and come to grips with the reality of their illness. This is especially critical for persons of colour or racial minorities. According to some theorists there exists a dualism in the character structure of minorities such that they are constantly struggling with the twin realities of pragmatic survival and transcendence or hope for a better world. This dualism is a psychological adaptation which allows such persons to adapt and persevere in a society which devalues them because of their skin colour (Chestang, 1974). According to dual personality theorists, at any given moment either aspect of the personality may be dominant dependent on the perceived threat from the environment. Being an AIDS victim is likely to tip the balance toward extreme despair and withdrawal; guilt, shame, anger, rage, hopelessness and powerlessness may constitute their psychological response rather than those of hope or transcendence.

These are critical factors in the prevention of AIDS. Despairing persons are not likely to be cooperative with authorities. There is a parallel in that gay and bisexual men, under the duress of the stigma of the fear of AIDS have grown more circumspect about revealing their sexual orientation due to attacks and hate campaigns directed toward them by reactionary groups (Batchelor, 1984). Increased public censure and reactionary laws based on racial and homophobic fears could succeed in isolating and alienating a substrata of AIDS victims (minorities) whose cooperation is sorely needed to control the spread of the disease. It appears clear that one of the major goals of this epidemic has to be prevention and this is tied to voluntary compliance with health regulations. Education remains the only weapon with any degree of efficacy in the war against AIDS. Prevention is sought through dramatically curtailed and "safe" sexual activity and reduced drug abuse involving contaminated needles. These are tough habits to change and will require massive public education (Boston Globe Editorial, 1986). Hostile and angry public responses are assured of finding an echoing response among minority victims. Many will likely remain or drop out of sight as habits of a lifetime learned on the streets and on the margins of society will be hard to surrender. This is to the detriment of a public health effort which requires the voluntary cooperation of at-risk groups in order to halt the spread of AIDS, particularly among the asymptomatic and ARC groups who constitute an invisible but ever present risk. To paraphrase Brian Comella (1986) of the Boston AIDS Action Committee, the population we are trying to reach is isolated, somewhat antisocial and they do not use traditional treatment centers . . . we must go where they congregate, which we learn of through the grapevine. You have to talk to people one on one and try to enlist them in the process (quoted in Malone, 1986). We simply cannot rest comfortably on the assumption that the disease will be confined to the lowly and that social class will exist as an effective barrier to transmission.

SOCIAL WORK PRACTICE AND AIDS POLICY FROM A MINORITY PERSPECTIVE

In every instance, a social worker working with an AIDS victim, whether in a hospital setting, in an AIDS service organization, a self-help group, or through traditional services, is involved in an epidemiological milieu in which the nature of his/her practice is constrained by forces larger than the needs of the individual client. The scope of this practice involves a range of professionals representing a true bio-psychosocial team: physicians, psychiatrists, psychologists, psychiatric and infection control nurses, substance abuse counselors, and medical epidemiologists and social workers. In addition to working directly in the health care setting, the social worker may also be called on to connect victims of the disease with needed community resources, with family and friends, be involved in the planning for home health care, legal aide, transportation, social security, general assistance, and to act as advocate liaison to charitable organizations. These are routine transactions except in the nonroutine environment of an epidemic and this fact may place demands on the worker for which the worker may be poorly prepared by dint of training or experience. At the core of the worker's activity is a group of professional values which may or may not be serviceable in a hysterical environment involving questions on the order of: what is to be done for the individual AIDS patients and what are the best means to control the disease? These questions may produce conflicts in the worker over matters of individual rights versus public safety. The social work values which appear most challenged by the AIDS epidemic are:

1. The belief in the primacy of the individual.
2. The belief in the right of self determination.
3. The confidentiality of client information.
4. A belief in a fair and equitable distribution of resources and services without discrimination, uninfluenced by race, ethnicity, sexual orientation or handicapping condition.

Social work values are not, perhaps, inconsistent with recent legal interpretations of current public health law which suggest that, with respect to the control of an infectious disease, and to protect the public health, states may use only those measures which are medically justified. Hence, although government may limit individual freedom to protect the public health, it must not use means that exceed those needed to achieve disease control goals. Means are selected only after a two step analysis of the circumstances surrounding the infection involving: (1) a medical judgement of the risk and mode of infection; (2) the selection of a response which considers psychological, sociological, political and economic factors (Yale Law and Policy Review, 1985). It is the latter step which is troubling to persons of colour and creates the potential of AIDS policies that are burdened by racism and homophobia. Owing to the prevalence in the U.S. of racial intolerance, sexual discrimination, mean spiritedness toward those residing at the bottom of the society, homophobia, and victorian moralism in matters of sex and sexually transmitted diseases a supreme effort will have to be undertaken to root out the prejudicial aspects of disease control policies and statutes.

Social workers, because of their ancillary role in AIDS control, generally under the direction of the medical profession, will find their value positions hard pressed to come to the fore. Claims for extraordinary methods of disease control in an epidemic are usually justified on the basis of the collective interests of society. The protection of individual and even group rights can be overridden by this priority. Confidentiality is threatened, as well, when the means of prevention might require the registration and monitoring of those posing a threat to public health and safety. How much self-determination can exist for persons who are already burdened by the exigencies of race, class, and gender and further debilitated by a life threatening illness? Lastly, homosexuality is illegal in half the states in the U.S. and drug abuse is illegal in all of them. As a result, a majority of AIDS victims are also statutory criminals subject to a variety of penalties. The protection of their rights is further complicated by this fact.

Value pragmatism rather than value rigidity may be the best stance for the profession in this climate. The field of social work will find itself having to cooperate and support positions for which our professed values provide little guidance to action. As a profession we must, however, support the principle of *voluntary compliance* as an appropriate method of controlling the AIDS epidemic. This takes into account the fact that coercion in the form of detention and quarantine are methods which appear to be ultimately doomed, forcing high risk groups into a kind of AIDS underground inaccessible to education or control. Secondly, we should support efforts to decriminalize the behaviour of victims of either homosexuality or drug addiction. Criminal penalties constitute unneeded coercion and can again lead to a reluctance to disclose behaviour and is counterproductive to the education/voluntary compliance strategy.

On balance, we may have to accept the registration and monitoring of those infected with AIDS. To do less would be to incur public ire and to risk the spread of disease by those unwilling or unable to comply with public health regulations. In extreme cases quarantine may be appropriate. These recommendations are made with the recognition that AIDS policies must be balanced carefully against the rights of the individual, that the victim is protected from the unnecessary intrusions of a fearful public. The profession must support programs to combat drug abuse while advocating the increased availability of clean, sterile hypodermic needles and condoms. Social work should, as well, support mandatory and voluntary screening with ample safeguards for privacy and confidentiality, as a means of identifying infected persons.

SOCIAL JUSTICE IN AIDS AND THE SOCIAL WORK ROLE

With regard to minorities and/or persons of colour, perhaps no other profession has given so much time and attention to the equal and just relations between racial and ethnic groups as social work and thus it has a critical role to play in enlisting those communities in self-determining efforts to eradicate the AIDS epidemic. The profession must seize this opportunity to bring its years of experience and insight to bear to protect AIDS victims against discrimination, to extend its services to them, to see that there is a just and equitable distribution of current and developing health and medical resources, and to see that the natural inclinations of a less than tolerant society do not hold sway to the detriment of the infected as well as the uninfected.

REFERENCES

Batchelor, W. (1984). AIDS: A public health and psychological emergency. *American Psychologist, 39*(11), 1279-1284.
Bickelhaupt, S. (October 19, 1986). Effect of AIDS on women outlined. *Boston Globe*, p. 40.
Boston Globe (October 6, 1986). Editorial: AIDS perception and reality. *Boston Globe*, p. 14.
Burris, S. (1985). Fear itself: AIDS, herpes, and public health decisions. *Yale Law and Policy Review*, 3, p. 479.
Chestang, L. (1974). *Character development in a hostile environment: An occasional paper*. University of Chicago. School of Social Services Administration.

Clark, M., McDaniel, A., Reese, M., Marshall, R., & Starr, M. (July 7, 1986). AIDS in the workplace: New ruling restricts protection for victims. *Newsweek*, 62-63.

Dieppa, I. (1984). Trends in social work education for minorities. In B.W. White (Ed.), *Color in a white society*, Silver Spring, MD: National Association of Social Workers.

Dowdle, W. (1986). AIDS: What is it? *Public Welfare*, *44*(3), 14-19.

Foreman, J. (October 6, 1986). Drug trial is opened to more AIDS patients. *Boston Globe*, 39.

Freedman, D. (1986). Wrong without remedy. *American Bar Association Journal*, *72*, p. 37, June.

Gonda, M. (May 1986). The natural history of AIDS. *Natural History*, *95*(5), pp. 78-81.

Greico, M. (November 15, 1985). Recommendations for preventing transmission of infection with HTLV-III/LAV in the workplace. *Morbidity and Mortality Weekly Reports*, 34, p. 682.

Ivey, H. (1985). AIDS. A presentation to the New York State Association of Black Social Workers' Conference, Syracuse, NY.

Jaret, P. & Nilsson, L. (June 1986). Our immune system: The wars within. *National Geographic*, *169*(6), 702-735.

Knox, R. (June 26, 1986). Scourge of AIDS spreads worldwide. *Boston Globe*, p. 1.

Knox, R. (June 26, 1986). AIDS readily transmitted from women to men, study shows. *Boston Globe*, p. 22.

Luehrs, J., Orlebeke, E., & Merlis, M. (1986). AIDS and Medicaid: The role of medicaid in treating those with AIDS. *Public Welfare*, *44*(3), pp. 20-28.

McLaughlin, L. (July 10, 1986). AIDS in Africa is spreading, seems impossible to check. *Boston Globe*, p. 19.

Malone, M. (October 6, 1986). Task force to educate drug users about AIDS. *Boston Globe*, p. 17.

Miller, J. (October 5, 1986). Prostitutes make appeal for AIDS prevention. *New York Times*, p. 8.

Morin, S. & Batchelor, W. (1984). Responding to the psychological crisis of AIDS. *Public Health Reports*, *99*(1), pp. 4-9 (January-February).

National AIDS Centre (1987). Personal communication.

Netter, J. (October 5, 1986). W.H.O. reports a sharp increase in AIDS cases. *New York Times*, p. 9.

O'Hara, J. & Stangler, G. (1986). AIDS and the human services. *Public Welfare*, *44*(3), pp. 7-13.

Press, A. & McDaniel, A. (March 16, 1987). A victory to AIDS victims. *Newsweek*, p. 33.

Seligman, J., Hager, M., & Springen, K. (June 23, 1986). Spreading the alarm about AIDS. *Newsweek*, p. 68.

United States Dept. of Health and Human Services (1986). *Coping with AIDS:*

Psychological and social considerations in helping people with HTLV-III infection. Washington, DC: National Institute of Mental Health, Dept. of Health and Human Services.

United States Department of Health & Human Services. Public Health Service Centre Disease Control. *Morbidity and mortality weekly report.* June 15, 1987.

Yost, P. (June 24, 1986). U.S. finds grounds for firing AIDS carriers. *Boston Globe*, p. 1.

Washington Social Legislation Bulletin. (January 13, 1986). The balanced budget and emergency control act of 1985, *29*(25), 97-100.

PART II: PRACTICE INTERVENTIONS

Counselling Issues
in Disclosure of
Sexually Transmitted Disease

Constance Lindemann

Sexually Transmitted Diseases (STD) are a major health problem in the United States with almost 20 million persons affected each year. About one-half of STD patients are under the age of 26. Untreated STD can lead to severe physical and mental health problems and even to death (Yarber, 1985). Scientists have classified more than 20 diseases specifically as STD (Yarber, 1985). Some of the most important are gonorrhea, syphilis, genital herpes, chlamydial infections, trichomoniasis, Pelvic Inflammatory Disease, and Acquired Immunodeficiency Syndrome (AIDS).

In all cases of STD, contacting the sexual partners of the clients who seek medical care and informing them of the possibility of infection is an important consideration. In the United States, case finding is the major public health method of controlling the spread of STD (Hanlon, 1964). This means contacting all known sexual partners of the client and letting them know that they are at risk and should obtain medical care for diagnosis and treatment.

A survey of social work literature from 1980 to 1986 from the

© 1988 by The Haworth Press, Inc. All rights reserved. *55*

subject index of *Social Work Research and Abstracts* (1980-1986) shows that social workers are involved in numerous aspects of sexuality. Some of these are sex roles, sexual abuse, sexual arousal, inhibition and dysfunction, sexual behavior, inequality, attitudes, education and communication, sexual relations, sexual preference, sex counselling and sexual harassment. Involvement in such a wide variety of sexual matters indicates that social workers have ample opportunity to impact on control of STD and have the appropriate background and experience. However, the same survey indicates virtually no attention to sexually transmitted disease. A computer based literature search by Carlton and Mayes (1982) indicates the same neglect. Involvement in such a wide variety of sexual matters indicates that social workers have ample opportunity to impact on control of STD and have the appropriate background and experience. In particular, in the area of behavioral education, social workers can play a significant role and it is with this objective that the article is concerned.

It reports on a one year demonstration project in a public health clinic that offered counselling to any STD patients who accepted the offer. Social workers were available during clinic hours to discuss and provide counselling on any matters that were brought up by the clients in these counselling sessions. Introduction of this type of project was possible because of the flexibility of STD programming. The Centers for Disease Control recognize that STD clinic services "must be appropriate to the special populations, disease problems and political settings of each program" and therefore encourages flexibility and diversity in clinic services among the various programs and locations (U.S. Public Health Service, 1985).

For this article the case notes for all the clients in that project were qualitatively analyzed for data on the disclosure of STD. The method that was used for the qualitative analysis was grounded theory (Glaser & Strauss, 1967; Glaser, 1978; Lindemann, 1974). This is a systematic method for coding, categorizing and analyzing qualitative data to generate meaningful concepts that can be used in practice and in further research. There were three reasons for the selection of this methodology. One was the lack of meaningful concepts as demonstrated by the paucity of literature on the subject. A second reason was the nature of the data. This methodology, unlike most others, lends itself to case notes that are idiosyncratic to the note taker. Since the purpose of the methodology is to generate concepts and categories from the data, there is no need for uniform categories to be present. Hence the methodology is particularly appropriate for clinical case notes that are recorded for the purpose of practice rather than for research purposes. A third reason is the recent recognition that

> social work's prevailing research paradigm is outmoded and restrictive, glorifies method (particularly quantification) over substance, and discourages contributions by practitioners. The profession must generate knowledge that is more relevant to the practitioner and more applicable to the important problems with which it is and will be confronted. (Pieper, 1985)

Although there are variations in case finding from clinic to clinic, at the one where the data for this study were collected the clients' first contact was with the Disease Intervention Specialist (D.I.S). The D.I.S. at this clinic took responsibility for case finding in those cases which would have the most serious consequences, such as congenital syphilis. For other cases the person who sought medical care was expected to take responsibility for contacting his or her sexual partners. There were a number of reasons why an STD patient failed in this responsibility. Analysis of the case notes indicated six factors which included lack of information about STD, lack of awareness and understanding of the need for disclosure, apprehension about the disclosure, avoidance of disclosure, client reaction to the prospect of disclosure and their anticipation of the partner's reaction, and finally the actual reaction of partners. The purpose of this paper is to discuss these factors in order to provide a basis for effective counselling that will facilitate disclosure of STD to sexual partners.

NEED FOR INFORMATION

The client may lack information about STD. Information should be provided about the symptoms, prevention and treatment of STD and about how it is transmitted. Often the client is too upset to absorb the information initially when it is offered by the D.I.S. who first sees the client. Clients can therefore benefit by follow-up repetition and clarification from a social worker. Additional information may be needed as more questions occur to the client after departure from the clinic. For this reason a telephone number should be supplied to the client or a future appointment should be set up.

Since 85% of STD occurs in persons between the ages of 15 and 30, a reasonable approach would be to use *STD: A Guide for Today's Young Adults* (Yarber, 1985). This guide cites the following outcomes for STD information and instruction: practice a lifestyle that decreases the chances of getting an STD, recognize symptoms of an STD, avoid exposing others if an STD infection is diagnosed or suspected, seek prompt medical care if an STD infection is suspected, follow a physician's directions if treated for an STD, get all sex partners to medical care if one has an STD, serve as a source of accurate information and advice on STD, be supportive and helpful to persons who get an STD, promote STD education, and research and health care. It should be noted that the latter two objectives pertain to professionals and are appropriate to social workers while all the other objectives are appropriate for social workers in practice with clients. Since this guide pre-dates the concerns with AIDS it should be supplemented with the Surgeon General's Report on AIDS (U.S. Department of Health and Human Services 1985).

Social workers traditionally have little or no education and training in this area and there is a need to develop courses and modules in basic social work curricula and in continuing education programs that incorporate this information, such as the courses and workshops outlined elsewhere in this special edition.

AWARENESS AND UNDERSTANDING

In many cases the client may not be aware of the necessity and importance of disclosing the disease to sexual partners, and of the possible serious consequences to them when the disease is not detected in its early stages. This is especially true for female sexual partners. Gonorrhea, for example, reveals symptoms in only 50% of females compared to 90% of males (Barlow, 1979). Therefore, 50% of women have the disease without symptoms which would ordinarily motivate them to seek medical care. Complications such as pelvic inflammatory diseases, sterility, or danger to the babies of pregnant women and potentially fatal infections may result from undetected and untreated STD (Frankfort, 1972).

Clients may be willing to tell their partners, but need techniques for such disclosure. In their words, they are "worried about what to say" and "how to tell their partners." Ho (1980) offers a number of strategies that may be applicable to this situation. One is simple straightforward advising which is appropriate "when experiencing a temporary crisis situation . . . (and) is used with the assumption that the client is capable, willing, and ready to take the course of action" (p. 151). Advice should be clearly labeled as such. Another technique is the Empty Chair. In this technique "the worker uses an empty chair, which represents an absentee with whom the client has unfinished business" (p. 239). The client then moves to the empty chair and portrays the absentee person and imagines that person's responses. A third technique is Logical Discussion. This technique is valuable in exploring specific areas that may be barriers to disclosure. Modeling is another technique that can be used. In this technique "the worker serves as a model for the client to observe and to imitate" (p. 245). Still another technique is Rehearsal. This technique allows a social worker to help a client to anticipate "and react to" the future situation (p. 259). The Rehearsal technique which might include the social worker playing the role of the partner as the client rehearses the disclosure, helps the client bridge the "gap between learning obtained in the worker's office and the application of such learning in the client's actual life situation" (p. 260). For each of these techniques Ho provides the advantages and disadvantages and kinds of clients and situations for which each is appropriate.

APPREHENSION ABOUT DISCLOSURE

While a few people are not uncomfortable about disclosing the fact that they have an STD, most are apprehensive about disclosure. The difficulty or ease with which a person faces the prospect of disclosure is influenced by the attitude toward STD, personal relationships, other relationships such as those with professionals and family, and accidental disclosure.

The first of these, attitude toward STD, suggests that difficulty about disclosing the disease may derive in some part from the reaction toward the disease itself. Some people are very upset about it while others are not at all troubled. Those who are not troubled may have a casual attitude toward STD. For them it may be in the same category as any other illness needing detection and treatment, and there is no concern over any negative connotations of the disease. In the words of one client, "if you get it, cure it." The data indicate that those who are upset about having the disease may be influenced by connotations of shame or social stigma attached to STD or may be upset at the fact that their sexual activity is disclosed. Attitudes toward the disease may also be influenced by repeated episodes of STD. In some cases repeated episodes are particularly upsetting because of clients' perception that it is the consequence of a dysfunctional behavior pattern. These attitudes affect the ability to talk about the disease to any sex partners. Information and counselling are needed to overcome such reactions. Counselling approaches may include interpretation which "brings new facts or rearranges existing facts so that the client may see his (or her) behavior in a different light" (Ho, 1980, p. 147); reflection of feeling where the worker expresses the "underlying attitudes of the client" thereby providing the client with the "opportunity to observe more objectively (his or her) own feelings" (Ho, 1980, p. 186); ventilating, which encourages a client to express feelings underlying the attitudes; and universalizing, where the worker "uses the commonality of human experiences" to help the client cope with the problem (Ho, 1980, pp. 209-211).

A second factor influencing disclosure is that of personal relationships. A full range of personal relationships are represented by the clientele of a clinic for STD, from those who have exclusively single-sex episodes with a number of different partners to those who have long-term continuing relationships with a single partner with or without marriage. The clientele also includes people of all sexual preferences. In the case of long-term relationships, the STD is contracted in an occasional sexual episode outside the relationship. There are also casual single-episode relationships where there is no further contact between the partners and, therefore, no possibility of contacting sex partners. Even long term relationships with no outside sexual relationships may be represented, since it is possible that a dormant case of herpes or AIDS may be activated without outside contact within the recent past. In all these types of relationships there are those who can talk about problems and issues that affect the relationship, including sexual matters and STD, and those who cannot talk about such matters. Ability to disclose STD, then, ranges from easy to difficult. Disclosure is more difficult in long term, ongoing relationships than in short term relationships. Although there are exceptions, it appears that the more involved the relationship and the more important the partner, the more difficult it is to disclose the existence of an STD. Conversely, the more casual the relationship, the easier it is to disclose. For example, one client, a married man, was comfortable with telling extramarital sex partners, but was very anxious about telling his wife. Difficulty in disclosure exists in homosexual as well as heterosexual relationships. A gay man with a limited number of sex partners said he would have "a hard time letting them know." Difficulty in disclosing STD may also be compounded by status differences in the relationship. The partner with the lower status may find it more difficult to disclose STD to a partner of higher status. This was the case for an unemployed male client living with a woman who had two jobs. He felt that not only was he not contributing his share to the relationship, but he was adding an additional burden by introducing an STD. This constituted a barrier to disclosure.

The family is a third factor which impacts upon disclosure. Perhaps one of the most difficult disclosures is to the family, especially for those who are young and still living with their families. Disclosure to family is not usual and is most often avoided. This is possible because most of the States allow treatment for communicable diseases for minors, including STD, without parental consent. However, there are cases where disclosure to family takes place with or without agreement of the young person, precipitating a complexity of issues and problems. In one such case a private family physician disclosed the STD to the family of a young woman still living at home whose steady boyfriend and intended husband contracted STD as a result of a rare outside sexual episode. In this case the family insisted on the breakup of this relationship. The problem may have been due as much to the revelation of the sexual activity of the daughter as to the disclosure of STD, but the complex issues that were precipitated by disclosing the STD illustrate the problems of disclosure in families.

Fourthly, apprehension about disclosing STD is not limited to personal relationships and to the family. Difficulty also occurs in disclosure to friends and acquaintances, and even the professionals who are sought for diagnosis and treatment. Difficulty in disclosure to professionals may be due to fear of the attitude of professionals toward people with STD, which in some cases may have been caused by an actual negative experience with professionals in the past. This may be dispelled by subsequent positive experience with professionals. Difficulty in disclosure to professionals may cause delay in seeking diagnosis and treatment. One male client with a second episode of STD said it was still "hard to come to the clinic, but when you have to go, you have to go." Most often the concern with professionals is around the issue of confidentiality. This concern is expressed particularly by those clients who are themselves providing services in the community such as hairdressers who fear that their business will be affected by disclosure to patrons. Not only is it necessary to assure clients of confidentiality, it may also be necessary to provide community outreach on this issue, so that the reputation of the clinic for strict confidentiality is known in the community.

Concerns expressed about the clinic also centre around the issue of confidentiality, particularly about accidental disclosure due to the location and timing of services. A single-purpose clinic, where only STD patients are seen or special clinic hours when only STD patients are seen makes evident the purpose of the visit to the clinic. It could be possible, then, to be seen by an acquaintance or a patron. As one client puts it, "I'd feel weird if I saw someone I knew there." The optimum solution is a multi-purpose clinic at a site that includes all other medical services. In Great Britain, for example, "in the last ten or fifteen years there has been a trend away from this geographical separation of the clinic, and there are now several-purpose built clinics . . . designed as integral parts of new hospital complexes" (Barlow, 1979, p. 16). In the United States where most STD clients are seen at public health clinics the situation could be alleviated by community outreach which could provide information about the multi-purpose nature of the clinic and about the other services provided by the clinic that are not related to STD or to the traditional public health areas of maternal and child health the latter of which might pose a barrier to male clients.

AVOIDANCE OF DISCLOSURE

Many clients prefer to avoid disclosure and there are circumstances in which this is possible. This option may be preferred regardless of any difficulties or unusual behavior necessitated by the choice.

One situation in which this choice is possible is when STD is contracted during the temporary absence of a steady partner in a relationship. The client can be treated for STD and completely recover by the time of the partner's return. This choice is so desirable that in one case a client became angry and hostile toward the STD clinic because of a disruption in the inoculation schedule for syphilis. He contracted the STD while his partner was away and expected to be completely cured before her return. The disruption delayed his recovery. In this case, the possibility of avoiding disclosure was threatened and apprehension about disclosure resulted in unpleasantness for client and clinic. In cases of absent partners where recovery is not possible by the time of the partner's return, disclosure may be avoided by refraining from sexual contact until the condition is cleared. A client who was involved in relationship for five years with intermittent separations contracted STD during one of those separations and refrained from contacting his girlfriend until after the episode of STD was over. He gave her no explanation for his behavior.

Physicians may play a role in avoiding disclosure, particularly in the case of a married couple where the wife sees a physician for regular gynecology checks. When data from the case notes indicates that the husband has previously contracted an STD the physician may treat the woman for an STD without disclosing to her the nature of the problem.

Physicians may be affected by the same stigma and negative connotations of STD as are patients. In addition, there is a certain amount of professional stigma that can be illustrated by contrasting conditions in Great Britain and the United States. In Great Britain STD are a recognized clinical speciality. Because of the connection between STD clinics and hospitals, including teaching hospitals, the practitioners in the field receive constant professional feedback from other medical disciplines. By contrast, in the United States STD is not even part of the standard medical school curriculum, clinics are not attached to university medical schools and, therefore, not attractive to good physicians as a speciality, there is a minimal amount of post graduate education in the subject, and there is little opportunity for feedback from other medical disciplines due to the separation of STD clinics (Barlow, 1979). In this context it is not surprising that physicians may be uncomfortable with and lack experience and expertise in STD cases and may be prone to avoid the issue with their patients.

Avoidance of disclosure is sometimes accomplished by pseudo-disclosure. In pseudo-disclosure neither partner discloses information about the sexual activity that led to contracting the disease. In fact both partners may deny sexual contact outside the relationship. In cases such as this, disclosure occurs when one of the partners seeks medical care as a result of symptoms. Disclosure actually takes place and treatment is obtained for the sexual partner, but neither partner acknowledges responsibility for contracting or transmitting the disease. This may have a disruptive influence on the relationship, perhaps greater than in actual disclosure, since there is suspicion of deceit by both parties. Pseudo-disclosure may occur in both hetero- and homosexual relationships.

Many clients wish to avoid responsibility for disclosure entirely and want someone else to take the responsibility. They would prefer that a third party, the health department, take complete responsibility for contacting and informing sexual partners. Some would prefer that the issue of disclosure not even be discussed with them. Others might accept the discussion, but would be, as one young female patient said, "glad the clinic is contacting the guy I got V.D. from." This attitude of clients may affect their ability to disclose the disease to sexual partners. In cases such as this they may need information about public health and clinic policy as discussed above in order to facilitate disclosure.

CLIENT REACTION

In addition to general apprehension, there are some specific reactions by clients as well as expectations and apprehension of the partner's reaction to disclosure. Apprehension may range from none at all to severe degrees of apprehension that effect disclosure.

Clients are often concerned about the emotional or physical effect on the partner and about the welfare of the partner. A client may fear hurting a partner physically or emotionally. This may occur in hetero- or homosexual relationships. Fear of physical damage to a partner may be intensified by the youthful age of a partner. One man was concerned about transmitting herpes to his girlfriend because she was so young. In a marriage there may be concern about the effect to disclosure on the marriage, per se, as distinct from the spouse's feelings. There is the possibility of a marriage breakup as a result of the disclosure.

Apprehension often causes delay and there may be concern about the consequences of delay. In one such case, a patient's girlfriend was six months pregnant and did not know either about the extra sexual affairs of her boyfriend, or about the STD. Her exposure to STD had taken place some time ago and the delay of disclosure placed her and the baby at high risk. The client in this case had delayed disclosure because of apprehension, and then was apprehensive about both the disclosure itself and the delay. This may not necessarily mean that the transmitter of the disease does not care. It is more often fear of losing a lover or fear of the anticipated reaction of a lover.

In other cases, a client may not be apprehensive at all about disclosure, even if an adverse reaction is anticipated. In these cases the client may view the difficulty as the partner's inability to handle the problem. In most situations there is apprehension about both disclosure and the partner's reaction to it. The client's anticipation of a partner's reaction has an effect on the degree of apprehension experienced by the client. The client may anticipate that the response of the sex partner to news of STD will be matter-of-fact and have

confidence that the partner will "get over it." This kind of anticipated response would minimize apprehension about disclosing the
disease. On the other hand, anticipation of a negative reaction max-
imizes apprehension.

ACTUAL REACTION OF PARTNERS

Many people come to the clinic as a result of disclosure by a sex
partner who is a client at the clinic so that the actual reaction of
partners to disclosure was observed and recorded in the case notes.
The actual reaction of partners to disclosure varies, similar to that of
the clients, from total acceptance to total rejection. There may also
be denial or restimulation of previous problems. The reaction may
be congruent with that anticipated by the client or may vary from it
to one degree or another.

There are some cases where there is a positive reaction from the
partner who is contacted. This may occur when the partner is also
sexually active outside the relationship and accepts STD as a probable consequence of a sexually active lifestyle. Disclosure is then
likely to be accepted in a matter-of-fact manner. This was true of a
young woman who made it a practice to have routine monthly
checks for STD because she was sexually active. She discovered
STD during one of these monthly checks. Since she has been having an exclusive relationship with one person for the previous
month, she was able to identify him as the transmitter. She brought
him in to be checked when she came for her own medication. They
both accepted the situation in a matter-of-fact way since they were
both comfortable with a sexually active lifestyle with multiple partners.

In other cases, the reaction of the partner goes beyond mere acceptance and the situation is more acceptable to the recipient of the
disease than to the person responsible for transmitting the disease.
In one case, a young man who was very upset by "bringing V.D.
into the relationship" was actually consoled by a girlfriend who
accepted the situation without being upset. This may reflect the
traditional role of women who are taught to be consolers and to
smooth things over (Norman, 1980; Miller, 1976) or to the "boun-
daryless empathy" that characterizes the female sex role (Bard-

wick, 1971). In this situation, some counselling with the woman on recognizing and caring for her own needs may be in order as a preventive measure for the future.

In another example of positive acceptance a young engaged man who came to the clinic had contracted STD shortly before his wedding day. His fiancée, whom he brought in for a check-up, was very understanding. She was concerned only that the infection be cleared before the wedding day. A possible explanation for her attitude might be the traditional sexual double standard for men and women (Gordon, 1976; Lindemann, 1974; Rubin, 1976), manifested in this case by the acceptance of traditional bachelor life including the last fling or "raucous parties preceding marriage" complete with venereal disease (Brandt, 1985).

At the other end of the reaction continuum are negative reactions to disclosure. Women, especially in marriage, often feel that it has "cheapened" the relationship. They fear repetition: "if it happens once, it will happen again." They may be concerned with the length of time it will take "to forget" and return to normal attitudes toward the spouse. They may even consider dissolving the marriage. Often it is as much the revelation of the extra sexual relationships, as the disclosure of the STD itself, that causes a more negative reaction. In one such case, the reaction had severe consequences. A pregnant woman who sniffed paint to obliterate the pain of disclosure subsequently miscarried the pregnancy as a result of the paint-sniffing.

With some individuals there is denial of disclosure. Many women simply refuse to acknowledge the possibility that they are at risk of STD when they are informed by a sexual partner. This is possible since women often have no symptoms with an active case of STD. Their denial may have severely adverse consequences since pelvic inflammatory disease, sterility and danger to offspring of pregnant women are frequent complications of untreated STD. Denial may reflect the sexual alienation of women (Phelps, 1979) which suggests that they, because of the loss of power in a male dominated situation, become alienated from their own sexual feelings and experience and relate to a world of symbol and fantasy.

In some cases, disclosure of STD may restimulate other problems. Opportunity to talk to a counselor after disclosure may provide the chance to work through previous problems that occurred when there was no such counselling opportunity. This was the case of a young woman whose recent stillbirth was of more concern to her than her feelings about STD. Problems that are restimulated require attention. However, caution should be taken that the disclosure and the feelings about STD are not totally eclipsed. The restimulated problem has to be dealt with on the feeling level, but the STD requires some task oriented, present-time reality recognition and effort.

CONCLUSION

Disclosure of STD to sexual partners is an important issue in the control of STD. Often the responsibility for disclosure rests with the client. Case notes from a public health clinic that were analyzed by a methodology for qualitative data revealed a number of psychosocial factors that may contribute to difficulty in meeting this responsibility. These factors include lack of information about STD, lack of awareness and understanding of the need for disclosure, apprehension about the disclosure, client reaction to the prospect of disclosure and anticipation of the partner's reaction, as well as the actual reaction of the partner.

Social workers can play a significant role in facilitating the disclosure of STD. A number of specific strategies to deal with clients' difficulties with disclosure have been outlined which may facilitate its process.

BIBLIOGRAPHY

Bardwick, J. M. & Douvan, E. (1971). Ambivalence: The socialization of women. In *Women in sexist society*, V. Gornick & B. K. Moran (eds.), New York: Basic Books.

Barlow, D. (1979). *Sexually transmitted diseases: The facts*. New York: Oxford University Press.

Brandt, A. M. (1986). *No magic bullet, a social history of venereal disease in the United States since 1880*. New York: Oxford University Press.

Carlton, T. O. & Mayes, S. J. (1982). Gonorrhea: Not a second class disease. *Health and Social Work*, 7(4), 301-313.

Frankfort, E. (1972). *Vaginal politics*. New York: Bantam Books.

Glaser, B. G. & Strauss, A. S. (1967). *The discovery of grounded theory*. Chicago: Aldine Publishing Co.

Glaser, B. G. (1978). *Theoretical sensitivity*. Mill Valley, CA: Sociology Press.

Gordon, L. (1976). *Woman's body, woman's right*. New York: Grossman Publishing (Viking Press).

Hanlon, J. J. (1964). *Principles of public health administration*, fourth edition. St. Louis: The C. V. Mosby Co.

Ho, M. K. (1980). *Social work methods, techniques and skills*. Washington, DC: University Press of America.

Lindemann, C. (1974). *Birth control and unmarried young women*. New York: Springer Publishing Co.

Lindemann, C. (1983). Sexual freedom: The right to say no. *Social Casework*. *64*(10), 609-617.

Miller, J. B. (1967). *Toward a new psychology of women*. Boston: Beacon Press.

Norman, E. (1980). Sex roles and sexism. In *Women's issues and social work practice*, E. Norman and A. Mancuso (eds.). Itasca, IL: F. E. Peacock Publishers.

Phelps, L. (1979). Female sexual alienation. In *Women: A feminist perspective*, second edition. J. Freeman, (ed.), Palo Alto: Mayfield Publishing Co.

Pieper, M. H. (1985). The future of social work research. *Social Work Research and Abstracts*, *4*(21), 3-11.

Rubin, L. B. (1976). *Worlds of pain*. New York: Basic Books.

Social Work Research and Abstracts (1980-1986). Subject Index. v., 16-22.

U.S. Department of Health and Human Services, Public Health Service, Centers for Disease Control. (1985). *Guidelines for STD control program operations*. Atlanta, GA.

U.S. Department of Health and Human Services. *Surgeon General's report on acquired immuno deficiency syndrome*. Washington, DC.

Yarber, W. L. (1985). *STD: A guide for today's young adult*. Reston, VA: American Alliance for Health, Physical Education, Recreation and Dance.

Issues and Problems Confronting the Lovers, Families and Communities Associated with Persons with AIDS

William Rowe
Gerald E. Plum
Clarence Crossman

INTRODUCTION

A recent popular account of the Acquired Immunodeficiency Syndrome (AIDS) epidemic (*Newsweek*, November 24, 1986) provides the official projections for the next five years. According to that account 179,000 deaths and 270,000 cumulative cases will be reported in the United States by 1991. The article suggests that these projections probably underestimate the extent of the epidemic in that: (1) they do not include estimates of AIDS-Related Complex (ARC) (in most surveys there are ten times as many cases of ARC as there are of AIDS); (2) the projections are based on estimates of the current extent of the epidemic. It is assumed that only those *already* infected with AIDS will be infected by 1991.

According to *Newsweek*, it is more likely that by 1991 approximately 5 million Americans will be carrying the AIDS virus and 60,000 Americans will die from the virus each year. While the authors are reluctant to promulgate statistics of a popular source that may be somewhat sensationalized, it would seem that regardless of which set of figures one uses to estimate the extent of the problem, the AIDS Epidemic remains underestimated in terms of its impact.

© 1988 by The Haworth Press, Inc. All rights reserved.

The figures themselves do not relate the extent of human anguish and suffering that will be felt by different members of the population. Information from the Shanti Project in San Francisco showed that as early as September 1983, for each person with AIDS (PWA) interviewed, there were more than two lovers, friends or family members who were also counselled (Morin and Batchelor, 1984). Unless prevention and treatment of the infection is forthcoming, it is difficult to believe that any health practitioner will not be involved in providing service to either the PWA or someone closely associated with him or her.

The purpose of this article is to alert practitioners to some of the issues that will be confronted by the lovers, families, and communities associated with the virus carrier. In this work the PWAs are limited to gay and bisexual men. In discussing families, both the family of origin, that is, parents and siblings of the homosexual male, and the acquired family, that is, the wife and children of the bisexual PWA are identified.

It has been helpful to utilize the distinction of induced versus rekindled issues made by Shernoff and Bloom (1985). The authors have found it additionally useful to add the notion of compounded issues. Issues or problems that are induced originate with the diagnosis of AIDS of the PWA. That is to say, the issue or problem has not existed before nor would any issue or problem exist in the absence of the diagnosis. Rekindled refers to problems or issues that existed in the past, have found some resolution, and are not re-encountered as a result of the diagnosis. Compounded issues or problems refer to situations where the diagnosis of the PWA interacts with an existing, manifest or latent pathology within the individuals or groups associated with the PWA.

To date, most contributions to the literature have been concerned with the problems and issues of the PWAs themselves. Little information is currently available regarding the impact of the AIDS epidemic on the lovers, families and the gay community. The information in this paper has been obtained from personal experience with the lovers, families and friends of PWAs, and from professional experience with clients who have been directly or indirectly affected by AIDS.

ISSUES FOR LOVERS OF PWAs

The issues that arise for two gay men in a primary relationship when one of them receives an AIDS-related diagnosis are obviously complex. The reactions to a life-threatening illness, that can be expected within any spousal relationship, can be anticipated within a gay male relationship. Those dynamics are intensified by the fact that sexual intimacy holds the potential for transmitting the virus between the two partners. The possibility of infection has created severe barriers to the sharing of intimacy between some lovers. In some instances the lover may develop an irrational generalized fear of the PWA himself

There is immense frustration felt by lovers who have used safe-sex precautions, but discover that they did not do so soon enough to prevent infection. That frustration can also be felt by gay men who choose to enter monogamous partnerships as an effort to avoid infection only to discover they have brought the virus and subsequent illness into the relationship with them.

It is common practice for medical practitioners to test the lover of a PWA for the presence of Human Immunodeficiency Virus (HIV) and for immunodeficiency on an ongoing basis. Feelings of anger and guilt can be evoked by these tests whatever their results. If the tests indicate that the lover of the PWA has not been infected, then the lover may well feel guilt and the PWA anger that one of them is threatened by death and one is not. If the testing indicates that the lover has been exposed to the virus, anger and guilt can be evoked by shared or private speculation as to whether one partner has infected the other.

The relationship bonds may not be strong enough or the partners may not be mature enough to withstand such emotional tension. There have been instances of lovers who out of terror and anger have forced PWAs and their belongings onto the street. Partners have also drifted away from each other as the emotional toll involved in confronting the illness and the fear around acts of sexual intimacy becomes too much to bear.

The lover may experience resentment over feeling compelled to remain in the relationship out of moral obligations. This would be particularly true where the diagnosis is compounded with existing problems within the relationship. In such cases the lover may experience both relief and guilt with the death of the PWA.

The lover under the stress of the dying process and out of a need to protect himself may be compelled to leave the relationship. This abandonment may induce feelings of intense guilt that would be difficult to resolve in the absence of the PWA.

Occasionally the PWA isolates himself from his lover. A couple affected by AIDS can also isolate themselves from friends and community involvement. PWAs have made statements about lovers such as, "He is better off without me," or "I could not bear to cause his death," and have subsequently withdrawn from a lover. This withdrawal is distressing to a lover who wishes to maintain intimacy and support. Couples who experience an irrational sense of contamination or an apprehension about the responses of others may isolate themselves from friends, family and community.

It appears common for couples to withdraw and test the sincerity and caring within their support systems by waiting for others to take the initiative to reestablish contact. It is important that the others meet this test in order that a supportive network be established for the lover both during the PWA's illness and following his death.

The position of the lover of a gay male with AIDS can be a vulnerable one in relation to the support systems that more easily deal with heterosexual couples. If the relationship between the lover and the legal family of a gay man with AIDS is not a positive one, the distress to the lover can be overwhelming. It is possible for a family to legally exclude a same-sex lover from information and decisions about health care and medical status, from funeral arrangements, from the estate of the PWA, and from shared possessions. It is even possible for family members to contest wills in which the lover is beneficiary or in which particular funeral arrangements are specified. There is grave indignity and an intensified sense of loss experienced by a lover whose partnership with a PWA is not respected.

Happily, there are some instances of lovers sharing positive, supportive relationships with families of gay men with AIDS. Often there is a tacit agreement to be cooperative and civil during the time of illness and death, with no intention of maintaining a relationship once the funeral is over.

The lover's access to his ill or dying partner as well as to information and decision-making is dependent on the sensitivity of health care professionals, because such a partnership has no legal status. A social worker in a health care setting can take the opportunity to act as advocate and help alleviate the tension and ill-treatment a lover of a PWA may be experiencing in relationship to health care workers or the family.

Partners, individually or conjointly, often wish to receive counselling support, but may assume that there are no helping professionals who would be open to their relationship and their particular health crisis. Even if they believe that counsellors do exist who are open and nonjudgemental, the task of distinguishing such persons from those who are not, can seem too formidable to undertake. Currently there is a pressing need for information about gay-positive, AIDS-informed therapists.

The loss and sense of aloneness felt after the death of a partner can be magnified by a gay man's fear that other men will not want to become involved with him. The grieving partner will need support when he initiates sexual and romantic involvement, and particularly if he does experience the rejection and fear of others. If the lover of a PWA has not disclosed his lover's diagnosis to family, friends or workmates, the resulting isolation and self-protection will add significantly to the emotional assault on his well-being. If the lover has not disclosed his own homosexuality, the isolation and self-protection will consume even more emotional energy. He will not be able to adequately explain the resulting change in his behaviour and functioning. The isolation will be permeated by a fear of further losses: loss of job, friendship or family ties. Ventilation of the surviving lover's fear, frustration and grief with a supportive person is crucial.

In light of the difficulties and adversity previously identified, it must be noted that some gay male lovers face AIDS and death with profound intimacy and dignity. These men provide inspiration and invaluable modelling for all persons facing crises in life and love.

ISSUES FOR THE FAMILY OF ORIGIN

This section identifies some of the issues faced by the family of origin, that is, the parents and siblings of PWAs. According to Nichols (1983), the emotional reactions of the PWA to the diagnosis of AIDS are the same as those described by Kübler-Ross in dying patients. These emotional reactions include shock, guilt, denial, fear, anger, sadness, bargaining, acceptance and resignation. According to Nichols, while the emotional reactions are the same, those of the PWA are more intense and labile. It may also be stated that the emotional reactions of the family of the PWA are similar to those of the family of the dying person — again are more intense and labile and also more mixed and ambivalent than those generally found in the families of a dying patient. In some cases the intensity of these mixed and ambivalent feelings appear to force a polarization in an attempt to resolve the intense distress caused by the diagnosis; for example, some parents express anger and not the hurt and loss, while other parents may express the hurt and loss but never appear to express any anger.

Predicting specific reactions on the part of families is difficult. The family's reaction is in fact a composite of the reactions of the individual members who may differ greatly in the quality of their responses. A number of factors seem to influence the reactions of family members. Among those factors are the degree of awareness of the PWA's gay lifestyle, the extent of homophobia experienced by different family members and the stigma attached to both a gay lifestyle and AIDS, the degree of status consciousness in the family, the intensity of the emotional reactions and the specific personality characteristics of different family members. In addition, the responses will be modulated through the values, beliefs and attitudes of individual family members. The worker's interventions will be different if the family has had prior knowledge of the PWA's gay lifestyle than if the information of the lifestyle is communicated with the diagnosis. In the former case the worker may reaffirm the previous defenses, strategies or modes of coping as opposed to having to identify these modes. For some families the initial stages of denial may be twofold, that is denying the illness and death and, at the same time, denying the PWA's homosexual lifestyle. In such cases, the problems faced by the parental family are induced by the diagnosis. For families that have been well aware of the PWA's homosexual lifestyle, the diagnosis rekindles many of their original concerns. For both families it appears that shock and denial are frequently intense and of long duration. Specific dysfunctional personality characteristics of individual family members when rekindled or compounded by the AIDS diagnosis serve as yet another source of variation in reaction. For example, a narcissistic parent with a high level of attachment and boundary problems may find it impossible to move beyond their own sense of loss, develop a variety of physical complaints and come to focus more on their own mortality than the illness and death of their son. The role played by the PWA in the family will also serve as another source of variation in reaction or response.

One cannot overestimate the impact of the stigma associated with a gay lifestyle and AIDS on the grieving process. The stigma attached to AIDS magnifies the stigma attached to a gay lifestyle. As a result the impact on a highly status-conscious family can be devastating. One grieving parent who was fairly accepting of his son's lifestyle shared his view that it must be much easier for a parent who loses his offspring in combat. While this parent believed that his son's own lifestyle, and indeed death displayed remarkable courage, it was difficult for him to feel that it was a noble death. Thus the parent may feel shame over the nature of his offspring's death and it becomes difficult, if not impossible, to share feelings and thoughts with others. This variable is probably significant in preventing many friends, lovers and family members from seeking therapeutic assistance. Again, even the most accepting non-gay parent will have some degree of homophobia and many have difficulty in accepting specific sexual acts that are part of a gay lifestyle and the transmission of AIDS. The difficulty in this area compounds the difficulties in sharing one's sense of grief. The possibility of a parent of a PWA turning to others for comfort or solace can be made difficult by the extent of homophobia experienced by others.

All of the above factors, and the list is not exhaustive, taken singularly can contribute to the variations in reactions and responses. When one considers the interaction of these factors, one begins to appreciate the varied and idiosyncratic reactions that are possible.

Having discussed the sources of variation in response and having alluded to the difficulty in anticipating specific reaction, it is still possible to identify some general issues and areas of concern for the family that have a high probability of occurrence. Among these are the process of grieving, reflections on parenting practices, crises of values and beliefs, stresses within the family and the reactions of siblings.

It may be that the overall task of the family is to achieve some resolution for their grief and loss and that other issues are variations on this task. While grieving may be too apparent to require identification, it is important to alert the worker to the fact that most of his/her work will take place within the context of grieving and that he/she must be prepared for intense feelings of loss and anger, as well as prolonged states of confusion among family members who do not impose structure through polarization or other means. Knowledge of the diagnosis and awareness of attempts of finding effective treatment will sometimes result in intense feelings of hope that the PWA will live until appropriate treatment is found. For many families, on the other hand, there is elicited a natural response to protect and nurture which is imposed on a strong sense of hopelessness and helplessness. This desire to protect can subsequently cause the PWA to experience a variety of emotional reactions toward the parent, hence demonstrating the complex interactive impact on families.

While perhaps the exception of suicide, it is difficult to imagine another form of death that forces reflections on parenting practices to as great an extent as the death of the PWA. Even the most accepting and liberal non-gay parent probably has some reservations about the relative value of his/her offspring's lifestyle. Parents of PWAs express vague guilt over their permissiveness, strictness, closeness, distance, acceptance, lack of acceptance or other qualities specific to their parenting style. A parent who has accepted his or her offspring's homosexuality may feel guilt around that acceptance, that is, he or she may feel that their acceptance has been instrumental in promoting their son's homosexuality and death. Conversely, the parent who has not accepted his/her son's lifestyle may feel guilt over that form of rejection and may feel that a general lack of acceptance is responsible for the homosexuality and death of the son.

One parent, somewhat sophisticated in psychological theory, speculated that his son was acting out his, the father's, projected feminine component. This speculation is an example of the convoluted extent to which some parents will reach for causality if not responsibility.

Such reflection may precipitate a crisis of values and beliefs. Parents may feel that their liberal, permissive attitudes are responsible or that their conservative, restrictive attitudes are at fault. One parent, who proclaimed to be an atheist, felt that his lack of belief was responsible for an unjust and severe punishment by God. Curiously, he also expressed his anger at the God he did not believe in. For parents of PWAs who practice fundamentalism, the challenge to values and beliefs may be alleviated by rejecting the son as well as his lifestyle and illness.

It is well known that there is an increased risk of family breakdown following the death of a family member and in particular an offspring. Such risks are even greater in the families of PWAs. There is a strong possibility that the diagnosis can be compounded with existing family problems. As parents feel the need to discover causality and responsibility, they may be blaming of the other parent. Problems in communication, closeness, affect expression and support will be intensified with the diagnosis. The different feelings that are expressed by polar types of families are probably experienced as polarities within the same family and the expression of these may be truncated or incomplete by virtue of the nature of the family and the diagnosis.

Parents, upon receiving information of the diagnosis, may not be available for other members of the family. In this case, the worker must be aware of and sensitive to the needs of other family members.

The loss of a member will change the structure and roles within the family. With the loss of one family member, it may be expected that some of the roles previously played by the deceased will be assumed by other family members. Given the complicated and value laden nature of the death, compensation and role assumption may not take place leaving the family with structural-functional deficits. Thus, the worker must be alert to the potential for the family and its members to regain a vital and meaningful existence in the absence of one of its members. Some family members have found it useful to work with groups providing assistance to PWAs and their families.

ISSUES FOR FAMILIES OF BISEXUAL MEN

It is difficult to obtain accurate data on how many bisexual men live a dual life as a husband and father and at the same time have a secret, sexually active homosexual life. Kinsey reported that close to 16 percent of single thirty-year-old men could be designated as bisexual (Kinsey et al., 1948). While it is unlikely that the percentage of married men who are bisexual is this high, informal reports from the gay community suggest there is a substantial group of men that fall into this category. The risk of contracting AIDS is greater for many in this group since they are more likely to frequent the parks, bars and baths in a quest for anonymous sexual contact. When such an individual is diagnosed with AIDS, the ramifications for his wife and children are significant and complicated. While there is some similarity in the factors that influence the reactions and responses described in the parental families of PWAs, there are a number of unique factors involved in the family of the bisexual male.

For many, the diagnosis results in a dual discovery for the family. First, is the frightening reality that the man has a contagious terminal disease, and second, that he has been involved in homosexual activity. Because of this, the normal emotional reactions to discovery that the father in a household is terminally ill are confounded. An immediate question that is raised for the spouse is her own risk of infection. To have been placed at such risk by her husband's sexual infidelity is an enormous psychological shock for most women. The resulting anger and hurt tend to be immobilizing at a time when all of the wife's emotional resources are needed to deal with the impending loss.

For most spouses their anger and hurt tend to vacillate between two polarities. One is directed at their husband, related to the betrayal of trust and the assumed irresponsibility— "How could he just go have sex with anyone?" The other is directed at themselves for being unaware and naive—"For ten years, he said he spent Saturday afternoon at the library." In some situations spouses wonder if they did not somehow "push" their husband into the gay world by being in inadequate sexual partner.

The children of the PWA also have a difficult dual adjustment upon learning of their father's diagnosis. They too must juxtapose their feelings related to the impending loss with their feelings of shame and anger. Most attempt to maintain secrecy about the AIDS diagnosis, but feel conflicted when friends and relatives offer support and condolence. Many teenage children have an especially difficult time because of their struggles around their own sexual identity.

Both the wife and the children face the loss of their previous social identity when the reality of the diagnosis becomes known. Even if friends and neighbours do not comment, many families report feeling like social pariahs; some family members stop attending church; avoid normal social involvement; and/or conspire to maintain confidentiality regarding the diagnosis or cause of death. In some cases the husband is sent to a different city for treatment. In one case a family decided to forego an insurance claim rather than allow the death certificate to be seen by the office staff.

One of the unique difficulties faced by the family of the bisexual PWA is that the expected emotional confusion accompanying the loss is compounded by having no precedents to serve as guidelines. Normally, family survivors take some solace in the fact that the feelings they are experiencing are similar to what they have observed in others. Whereas family members of PWAs have exclaimed, "I don't know what to feel—I don't know what is right."

In most situations where a man has been living a dual life, there has been some degree of accommodation in the family dynamics. This may be conscious, but most often it is unconscious, or at least out of awareness. Some men have been emotionally unavailable for their wife and children all along and as a result, the discovery of their situation is less emotionally intense for their family. Such families may, however, get in touch with feelings of neglect and intense anger about being emotionally "ripped off" in terms of a "normal" family life.

Some PWAs demand rigid adherence to strict moral and social codes from their families in what appears to be a reaction formation against the moral implications of their own dual life. When faced with the hypocrisy and incongruence of the man's behaviour, these families react with outrage at the "demanding tyrant" who has not lived by his own rules. For other families this new "problem" may be added to a list that may include, depression, alcoholism and verbal and physical abuse. The families in these situations sometime display a mixture of anger, self-recrimination and resignation when confronted with the diagnosis of the PWA.

GAY AND LESBIAN COMMUNITY

AIDS has had a profound impact on the gay and lesbian community. For many gays and lesbians there are overlapping areas of interest and concern. These overlapping areas and the social affiliation often observed is what is referred to as the gay and lesbian community. It has called forth a maturity in the face of crisis that marks another step in the coming of age of a people. It has also caused much emotional distress and "dis-ease" which could be alleviated in part by professional support. Individuals and couples seeking counselling are likely to name fear of AIDS as a concern with which they need help. AIDS has influenced how the gay and lesbian community is viewed by groups and institutions in society. AIDS has also influenced how segments of the gay and lesbian community interact with each other.

The increased visibility of death and dying has had profound effects on the gay and lesbian community. Most senior members of the gay and lesbian population are invisible, even within the community itself and until this point, the community has not had to face significant numbers of its members dying. Facing death and dying normally involves a reexamination of the values by which one lives; the AIDS crisis has predictably inspired an assessment of gay and lesbian liberation and lifestyles by its participants. Issues of spirituality, intimacy and friendship, political activism, and sexual expression are being readdressed in light of the AIDS threat.

Any crisis causes a great deal of distress and dysfunction. It can be expected that facing the fact that practices which were associated with sexual liberation have become a possible means of death results in frustration, demoralization and anxiety.

Some members of the community have radically altered their sexual practices based on fear rather than the deliberate learning of safe-sex practices. Practices born out of fear rather than deliberate choice result in diminished fulfillment and consequent loss of self-esteem. Some gay men experience a rekindling of self-hate and homophobia which they had thought had been irradicated. As a result, some members get out of the community they once found to be a support, and those with a bisexual capacity may even attempt to pursue heterosexual lifestyles and relationships. Some men have become fatalistic about the risk to themselves and others and make no changes in their sexual behaviour.

Rifts within the community can deepen if particular members wish to distinguish themselves from others they consider to be more at risk. For example, monogamous couples may criticize those people who are promiscuous and those who practice more conventional sexual activity may look askance at individuals who are involved in less conventional activity. Additionally, lesbians may criticize what they perceive to be risky gay male behaviour.

Another outcome of the AIDS crisis is a tendency to become disillusioned with particular expressions of sexual liberation and to return to sexual mores which, at one time, had been considered oppressive. With this shift in mores it becomes easy to accept negative descriptions of gay men and lesbians as narcissistic and immature.

One of the irrational sentiments that has reemerged during the AIDS crisis is that any disease contracted through sexual activity is deserved and any pleasure we experience must be paid for.

There are several groups of people within the gay and lesbian community who could benefit from professional support. There is a large number of "worried well" who are experiencing significant "dis-ease" because of the threat of AIDS. There are many gay men who have tested positive to the HIV-antibody test and are distressed about their potential for developing AIDS-related illnesses. There are leaders in the community who have taken on the added responsibility of responding to the AIDS crisis and volunteers who are devoting large amounts of their time and energy to AIDS projects and committees, who need care and support to maintain their own well being. In addition there are the friends, frequently of long standing, who will experience considerable grief and loss with the illness and death of a valued companion.

Not all of the impact on the gay and lesbian community needs to be viewed as negative. The crisis has enhanced a maturation and growth process both within the individual members and the community as a whole.

Sexual liberation can inspire sophisticated ethical decision-making and the presence of AIDS requires even more sophistication. It takes a significant degree of moral maturity to say that certain sexual acts are risky because of the possible transmission of a virus without saying that those sexual acts are wrong in and of themselves. The AIDS crisis has provided the opportunity for gay men to explore expressions of intimacy that are not explicitly sexual and sexual acts that are not explicitly genital. There is also a maturity in the way in which many segments of the community have cooperated in response to the AIDS threat: to form and finance grass roots AIDS projects and committees; to disseminate information about the disease and safe-sex practices; to provide support for those directly affected by AIDS. There is a renewed cooperation and appreciation between lesbians and gay men who make the effort to share energy and resources.

The gay and lesbian community is being viewed and is learning to view itself as an invaluable resource and pathfinder for society as a whole. The existence of the community in relationship to governments has taken on a new validation with the funding of AIDS projects and committees initiated by gay men and lesbians, and by governments seeking advice concerning policies and decisions from the gay and lesbian community. These projects and committees provide information and services to the general public and to health care and helping professionals. As a result there has been a growing appreciation of the way in which the community demonstrates its maturity and concern and a new understanding of gay and lesbian lifestyles.

The coming out process is a valuable experience for building resources with which to deal with loss. Coming out, accepting and disclosing one's homosexual orientation has been described as a grieving process and the stages of grieving as outlined by Kübler-

Ross also identify the coming out process (Fortunato, 1982; Massiah, 1985). The gay and lesbian community has considerable resources and experience in coping with loss that can be an invaluable resource to the social work practitioner.

ISSUES FOR THE WORKER

Most helping professionals are as yet unprepared to deal with the kinds of issues their clients must face related to the AIDS health care crisis. Both the scope and the long-term effects of the epidemic are as yet undetermined. In the absence of substantiated methods of intervention or even an accepted treatment protocol, social workers must respond to the needs of their clients with a mixture of conventional wisdom and necessary innovation. The following recommendations may prove helpful:

1. The worker must accept the extent of the epidemic and the necessity for a mature and compassionate response. If the worker does not currently have an individual in their practice who is in some way related to a person with AIDS he/she is likely to in the near future. Currently there is a need for workers to communicate both their readiness and willingness to respond to PWAs and persons involved with PWAs. This knowledge can be significantly reassuring for persons who feel isolated and stigmatized by virtue of their relationship to a PWA.
2. The worker must attain accurate and current information about AIDS and AIDS-related issues. One of the most commonly reported frustrations of people related to PWAs is the difficulty in obtaining information. "Everybody seems to say something different" is a common complaint. Many clients will demonstrate an insatiable need for information. Some have reported becoming "obsessed with gathering every fact about AIDS." Individuals who feel that something has happened to them that is beyond their control can often restore some sense of control by becoming informed. The worker can be helpful to this process by providing accurate information and dispelling myths. Information should be gleaned from a variety of sources and corroborated where possible.

3. Most workers, as part of their training or during their first few years of practice, have had to access their attitudes and beliefs in order to control for hidden bias or prejudice in working with value-laden topics and non-traditional lifestyles. Workers must review their beliefs and feelings about homosexuality, promiscuity and family systems in order to be sensitized to the issues and accepting of the concerns that will be raised by their clients. Both the gay and non-gay worker need to become aware of damaging stereotypes that he/she may harbour regarding both gay and non-gay clients (Dilley et al., 1985). Because the material is value-laden and the client's responses are emotionally intense, the workers in a clinical relationship with individuals related to PWAs must cautiously review their countertransference. For example, the clinicians may find themselves urging their clients to focus on their anger when other feelings are equally present or simply join with their client in a state of helplessness and despair.

4. Self-help or mutual aid groups provide a curative experience of universality and sharing that is extremely valuable to this group of clients. Although a few such groups have begun in large centres, there is a need for their establishment and facilitation on a wide scale. The tendency for people to withdraw and isolate themselves following the loss of a loved one, when coupled with the stigma and shame associated with AIDS makes the establishment of such groups difficult. There are many people experiencing unattended suffering, a fact which calls for energetic and innovative efforts to provide individual or group support.

5. The worker must become knowledgeable about safer-sex practices for both high risk groups and the population in general. The experiences of sex educators has shown that moralistic or judgemental approaches are ineffective in contrast to matter-of-fact or eroticized methods (Presten, 1985; Gay Men's Health Crisis, 1986). Workers must take every opportunity to promote safer-sex practices.

A unique ethical issue is raised when working with clients who are antibody positive and have chosen not to inform their sexual partners. The worker must address the conflict between maintaining confidentiality and the protection of people at risk.

Hart (1986) stated that "the AIDS crisis may make the most significant impact on the delivery of health and human services since the Social Security Act of 1935." Social workers are uniquely equipped to respond to the issues and circumstances created by the AIDS epidemic. Where possible, workers must become active in AIDS committees, involved in the development of resources and the identification of gay-positive counsellors.

Finally, it must be recognized that working with PWAs and related persons is stressful and demanding and the potential for burn-out is very high. It is crucial that workers establish support groups or networks to help mitigate the accumulative strain that is inevitable.

SUMMARY

Given the scope of the existing AIDS epidemic and the projections for the next five years, social workers must accept that they will almost certainly be providing service for PWAs or persons related to them. In this article an attempt has been made to identify the issues and problems that confront the lovers, families and communities associated with PWAs. The information presented in this work derives from both personal and professional contacts with persons related to PWAs. The perceptions and recommendations presented are based on practice experience. It is necessary to follow up these clinical perceptions with the accumulation of objective data to help the worker identify additional areas of concern and formulate appropriate interventions.

REFERENCES

Dilley, J., Ochitill, H., Perl, M., & Valberding, P. (1985). Findings in psychiatric consultations with patients with acquired immune deficiency syndrome. *American Journal of Psychiatry, 142*(1).

Fortunato, J. (1982). *Embracing the exile.* New York: Seabury Press.

Gay Men's Health Crisis. (1986). *Educational package.* New York.

Hart, M. (1986). AIDS: The most significant impact on human services since the Social Security Act of 1935. Paper presented at Clinical Social Work Conference. San Francisco, 1986.

Institute for the Advanced Study of Human Sexuality. (1986). *Safe sex in the age of AIDS*. Secaucus, New Jersey: Citadel Press.

Kinsey, A. C., Pomeroy, W. B., & Martin, C. E. (1948). *Sexual behaviour in the human male*. Philadelphia: Saunders.

Massiah, E. (1985). Lesbian existence and coming out: A reason to grieve. Paper presented to the Annual Symposium, National Association of Social Workers. Chicago.

Morin, S. & Batchelor, W. (1984). Responding to the psychological crises of AIDS. *Public Health Reports*, *99*(5), 4-9.

Nichols, S. (1983). Psychiatric aspects of AIDS. *Psychosomatics*, *24*(12), 1083-1089.

Presten, J. (1985). *Hot living: Erotic stories about safer sex*. Boston, Mass.

Shernoff, M. & Bloom, D. (1986). The impact of AIDS on gay men: Treatment issues for the private practitioner. Paper presented at Clinical Social Work Conference, San Francisco, September 11-14, 1984.

Slaff, J. & Brubacher, J. (1985). *The AIDS epidemic: How you can protect yourself and your family – why you must*. New York: Warner.

Psychosocial Dimensions
of Genital Herpes:
A Case Study Approach

Carole Christensen
Tatiana Kitsikis

INTRODUCTION

The number of people suffering from genital herpes has reached alarming proportions in North America in recent years. The dramatic rise in the incidence of this viral infection has been referred to as the scourge of the 1980s. It has also been interpreted as punishment for the sexual liberation of the 1970s. An estimated 20 million people in the United States suffer from this disease (Drob & Bernard, 1986); Canadian estimates run as high as 50,000 new cases annually (Lawee, 1982). Although reactions in various professional communities have varied, it has been impossible for medical researchers and practitioners, as well as health care providers, to ignore the growing number of people seeking relief from the various symptoms associated with the disease. To date, considerable attention has been focused on exploring the transmission, diagnosis, and treatment of genital herpes; however, little is known about its psychological and social consequences. Social workers have, apparently, been slow to respond to the special needs of this client group, although they are often the first line of defense for sufferers. As professionals skilled in the provision of psychosocial treatment methods, social workers have a unique role to play in helping genital herpes sufferers.

This paper attempts to shed light on the range and determinants of personal reactions found among genital herpes sufferers. A case

© 1988 by The Haworth Press, Inc. All rights reserved. *89*

study approach is used to illustrate the participants' psychological responses and relationship concerns. Specific suggestions are made for incorporating interventive methods appropriate to aid clients afflicted with genital herpes.

In order to counsel clients effectively, social workers must have an understanding of why certain medical aspects of the disease may have psychosocial dimensions, particularly at a time when wide media coverage has given rise to a number of misconceptions.

SIGNIFICANCE OF MEDICAL ASPECTS OF GENITAL HERPES

Although social workers are not usually expected to counsel clients about the medical aspects of genital herpes, and a detailed discussion of the medical aspects of the disease is beyond the scope of this paper, it is important that helpers who are not medically trained should have a basic knowledge of the symptoms of initial and recurrent outbreaks, and possible complications. Familiarity with the disease process is essential in order to be able to distinguish between those having common reactions and those whose responses suggest the need for therapeutic intervention. Helpers must have an understanding and appreciation of why certain medical aspects of the disease may have psychosocial outcomes which can be more or less distressing.

First, it must be recognized that genital herpes is associated with social stigma. The Herpes Simplex Virus (Type 1) which causes cold sores is essentially the same as that which manifests as genital herpes (Type 2) (Hamilton, 1980); but the mode of transmission (usually through sexual contact) location, and associated consequences cause the latter to be classified as a sexually transmitted disease (STD). As noted by Gulas and Griffith (1984):

> There is, however, an unmistakable difference in our emotional reactions to the location of the viral attack founded on society's misconceptions and attitudes about certain parts of our bodies and the association of genital herpes with sexual activity. (p.3)

Second, the symptoms and their location may be a source of considerable discomfort and embarrassment. These include blister-like sores on the thighs, buttocks, anus, external and (in women) internal genitals; as well as muscle aches and pains, fever, and headaches. Although symptoms form a spectrum from mild to severe, they tend to be most severe during initial outbreaks.

Third, once contracted, the genital herpes virus is likely to recur, because there is no known cure able to rid the body of the virus. However, the drug Acyclovir (Zorifax) can be effective to lessen symptoms and hasten the healing process (Reichman, Badger, Mertz et al., 1984). Recurrence appears to be triggered by emotional stress, the menstrual cycle, and sexual intercourse (Sacks, 1983). Since the infection can be asymptomatic and, in women, internal (i.e., affecting the cervix or inner two-thirds of the vagina) it is not always possible to know how or when it was contracted.

A fourth medical factor with important psychosocial implications is that a number of potentially hazardous complications have, reportedly, been related to genital herpes. These include cervical cancer and risks to newborn infants delivered vaginally, during an active phase of the disease (Bettoli, 1982; Cuthbert, 1981).

Finally, the treatment of genital herpes often affects the life-style of those afflicted. Decreasing the amount of smoking and drinking, adequate rest, and extra attentiveness to personal hygiene and levels of stress are among the health care precautions many find helpful (Montreal Health Press, 1984, p. 29).

PSYCHOSOCIAL DIMENSIONS OF GENITAL HERPES

Social work is unique among the professions in its focus on directing helping activities toward enhancing the functioning of people in interaction with their environment. Moreover, social workers, especially those in medical settings, have an opportunity to play a significant role in meeting the psychosocial needs of patients. Well-informed social workers should, therefore, experience little difficulty comprehending the many psychosocial ramifications of genital herpes for afflicted individuals. As is true of most problems brought to social work practitioners, psychosocial responses to genital herpes are, apparently, determined by a number of personal, cultural, and societal variables.

Sociocultural Variables

Throughout modern history, North Americans have tended to have an ambivalent love-hate relationship with sexuality, rooted in religious teachings and remnants of a Victorian era morality. The rise in the incidence of genital herpes is occurring simultaneously with a return to more conservative attitudes and values. Consequently, many view the widespread outbreak of genital herpes as fitting punishment for over-indulgence in sexual activity. Those who have begun to have sex at a younger age, perhaps with a number of partners, and whose activities include oral-genital practices, are viewed by some as leading immoral lives. Moreover, the greater number of people choosing to marry later, or not at all, the high divorce rate, and the forming of liaisons solely for the purpose of sexual gratification represent relatively new phenomena. Many observers view the widespread fear of contracting genital herpes as related to societal conflict about recent changes in sexual mores (Gallagher, 1982). Jokes about genital herpes abound, and sufferers are often depicted in the media as promiscuous, immoral and contemptible. The anticipation of a negative response has made many herpes victims reluctant to disclose the fact that they are carriers of the disease. This adds both to the likelihood that the disease will be spread to unsuspecting partners and to the lack of adequate societal response to those already affected.

Psychosocial Variables

Individual psychological responses to genital herpes range from mild and temporary distress to severe and lasting emotional trauma. A number of factors determine haw an individual responds upon contracting the disease, including demographic factors, cultural background, interpersonal relationships, self-concept, and previous emotional adjustment.

With regard to demographic factors, area of residence (e.g., rural, small town, or urban environment) is an important consideration. Those living in rural or small town environments may have feel that they cannot possibly hide the fact that they have contracted herpes, or the circumstances under which the disease was contracted. Civil status (i.e., whether the individual is single or in a permanent relationship) and age are other factors having psychosocial implications. The disease most often strikes those who are young, at a time of life when they are least likely to be involved in long-term, committed relationships (Luby & Gillespie, 1981). Gender is an important demographic factor, since women are affected by concerns peculiar to their sex (e.g., infection of internal organs, possible complications during childbirth). Education plays an important, but sometimes contradictory role; depending on the accuracy and presentation of the information received (e.g., the degree of sensationalism in media reports) and the personal response of the particular individual, anxiety levels may be unduly raised (Gillespie, 1982). No evidence was discovered in the literature to suggest that emotional responses to genital herpes vary according to income level. Centers for the treatment of the disease appear to attract people from all socioeconomic backgrounds (Drob, 1984; Woodis, 1983).

Cultural aspects are an important consideration in pluralistic societies, such as Canada and the United States, those experiencing genital herpes infections come from many different cultural, ethnic, and religious backgrounds. The extent to which an individual who contracts an STD is stigmatized, ostracized, shamed, and socially isolated varies among people from different backgrounds. Psychological distress often adds to the individual's inability to accept the realities of the disease, and deters the seeking of medical help and emotional support. Women from backgrounds where females are expected to give the appearance of chastity before marriage fear being seen as less desirable mates should they reveal to a prospective partner that they have genital herpes. Those from some religious backgrounds may engage in sexual activity outside of marriage with ambivalence, and view genital herpes as punishment for immoral behavior. On the other hand, individuals holding hedonistic values may be disinclined to warn prospective casual partners, or to change a former way of life. The importance of the worker's taking a person's cultural or ethnic background into account in the assessment and treatment of psychosocial responses to genital herpes cannot be overemphasized.

The nature of the individual's interpersonal relationships becomes important once the disease has been confirmed and ethical issues must be dealt with (i.e., if, when, and how to share information about the disease with one's intimate associates). If trust and communication between partners has been poor previously, difficulties may be exacerbated by the need for open communication concerning the course of the disease. Uninformed lovers who contract genital herpes may be angry, or suspicious about a partner's fidelity. The need for communication leads some to achieve greater intimacy, but others feel compelled to remain in relationships longer than planned, feeling that the disease makes them less desirable partners. Those who have not developed intimate interpersonal relationships may feel particularly lonely if they have no close friends or relatives with whom they can discuss their feelings about having genital herpes. Some may decide to adopt celibate lifestyles, and tell no one. On the other hand, sufferers who are married, or in long-term relationships, may experience a loss of spontaneity or interest in sexuality (Drob, 1984).

With regard to self-concept, individuals with genital herpes may feel contaminated, dirty, ugly, damaged, or inferior, particularly when recurrence is experienced (Drob, 1984). Many fear rejection and permanently ruined lives. Although herpes does not preclude safe procreation, some may feel unfit to be parents. Low self-esteem may lead to internalization of the stigma associated with genital herpes, resulting in intrapsychic conflict. Since genital herpes often attacks young people whose psychosexual development is in a state of flux, it may trigger or worsen conflicts concerning sexuality, intimacy, and commitment (Luby & Gillespie, 1981).

Depending on the individual's previous emotional adjustment, some or all of the following feelings may be experienced, to a greater or lesser extent, and lasting for shorter or longer periods: shock, anger, depression, fear and anxiety, isolation and loneliness, guilt and shame, self-pity and self-blame (Manne, Sandler, & Zautra, 1986). Individuals who have met and solved earlier crises and problem situations successfully are likely to make the adjustments necessary to cope with genital herpes without undue emotional stress. However, a significant minority may need professional help (Drob, 1984).

COPING WITH HERPES

Stages in Adjustment Process

Luby & Gillespie (1981) have outlined the following stages commonly experienced by genital herpes sufferers in the course of the natural adjustment process: (1) initial shock and emotional numbing; (2) real or imagined doubt over their diagnosis; (3) search for a cure and reassurance; (4) various degrees of feelings of isolation, loneliness, and self-doubt; (5) anxieties about contagion, childbirth, and interpersonal ethical issues raised by the disease; and (6) intermittent periods of depression brought on by recurrences.

Psychotherapeutic Methods

Most treatment methods known to social workers and other helpers have been used for clients with genital herpes. The appropriate treatment method varies, of course, according to the needs and responses of the individual client. Among the commonly used methods are: (1) information and counseling, aimed at clarifying misconceptions and adjusting to the realities of living with the disease; (2) cognitive therapy, to alter attitudes, distorted thinking, and perceptions (Greenwood & Bernstein, 1982); (3) psychodynamic psychotherapy, when the disease serves a psychodynamic or interpersonal function (e.g., the avoidance of intimacy); (4) group therapy, allowing the sharing of feelings, solutions, and ethical issues; (5) self-help groups such as Herpetic Engaged Living Productively (H.E.L.P.) (in the United States) and Research, Education and Assistance for Canadians with Herpes (R.E.A.C.H.) provide members a source of up-to-date information and sympathetic support (Woodis, 1983); (6) assertiveness training, for those needing to learn how best to disclose information about their condition (Drob & Bernard, 1983); (7) relaxation training seeks to diminish stress reactions believed to exacerbate the severity and frequency of outbreaks (Gillespie, 1982); (8) couple therapy, when conflicts engendered by the disease uncover latent relationship problems; (9) sex therapy, emphasizing behavioral techniques, for temporary impotence, orgasmic disfunction, or lack of desire.

Despite efforts of various individuals and groups to respond to the needs of those coping with genital herpes, there is a dearth of well-documented literature examining the psychosocial dimensions of the disease.

The experience of four people with genital herpes are presented below, in order to illustrate possible psychosocial effects of the disease.

CASE ILLUSTRATIONS

Based on the literature reviewed, a structured interview schedule was designed specifically for the purpose of eliciting responses relevant to the subject under consideration. The open- and close-ended questions covered: demographic information, the history of pertinent medical aspects of the disease, and psychosocial reactions to the affliction. In addition, one question asked how a professional social worker could be of help to herpes sufferers. A male and a female experiencing a first outbreak, and a male and a female with recurrences, were sought to respond voluntarily to the questionnaire. It was decided to limit the participants to those under 30 years of age.

Potential respondents were referred by nurses attached to infectious disease clinics in hospitals located in a Canadian metropolitan area. The nurses approached potential interviewees explaining the purpose of the study. Those who agreed and met the criteria were contacted and interviewed by the second author under conditions in which confidentiality was assured. Interviews were audiotaped and content analyzed.

Case #1 (First Outbreak)

Anne is a 28 year old, Caucasian French Canadian divorcee, who has lived with her 31 year old partner for one year. A 3 year old daughter from her marriage lives with her former husband. Anne is a secretary with a high school education, but is presently unemployed. She is from a Catholic background and "believes in God, but not in the dictates of the Church." Although she has had frequent yeast infections since becoming sexually active at the age of 15, her first experience with an STD or any chronic illness occurred when she contracted genital herpes one month ago. Before having the disease, stomach pains of unknown cause had already affected her sex life negatively.

The first outbreak of genital herpes was very painful, causing burning sensations when urinating and pain near the entry of the vagina, the primary area of infection. The outbreak subsided after one month. She "has no idea" how she contracted herpes, having only had sex during the past year with her current boyfriend, who does not have the disease. She never had oral herpes or engaged in oral-genital sex. Anne was shocked to learn that she had genital herpes, because she had believed that only the promiscuous get it. Other feelings included denial, disappointment, fear, and mild depression because of the incurable nature of the disease. Anne knows it is illogical, but feels jokes about herpes are directed at her. However, she has not found herpes as bad as she would have expected from media reports, which had led her to equate it with AIDS, or "the end of the world" before gaining accurate information. She stopped sexual intercourse due to the pain involved, and felt less pleasure and interest in sex. Prior to having genital herpes, she was "moderately active" (had intercourse twice a week) viewing sex as a necessary and exciting part of life. Problems achieving orgasm have always been present, but are worse since the herpes outbreak. She does not fear transmitting the disease since her only partner is aware of her condition. However, she has stopped the enjoyable practice of bathing with her daughter. No medical treatment has been used to combat symptoms.

Only Anne's boyfriend, who accompanied her to the doctor's office, knows that she has genital herpes, which she describes as "nothing you'd want to advertise." She tells her partner "everything," and describes him as a warm person who does not overreact. He was understanding and supportive, suggesting that they collect accurate information. In terms of intimacy and commitment, nothing changed. Should the relationship with her boyfriend end, Anne would feel obliged to tell her new partner that she has genital herpes, but would be anxious about his possible reaction. She fears that a break-up would mean living alone.

Professional support has been sought only from a clinic physician, who offered no reassurance, but coldly informed Anne that she had genital herpes, handing her a pamphlet. The nurse was more supportive. Anne wants medical treatment to relieve her pain, but feels no need for psychological help and had not heard of self-help groups for herpes sufferers. She could imagine seeing a social worker to help her cope with the situation if she broke up with her current partner, and had to face dating someone new. She also felt social workers had a role to play in disseminating accurate information.

Case #2 (First Outbreak)

Bruce is a 22 year old Black male from Trinidad, who has lived in Canada for 6 years. His fiancée remains in Trinidad. He is a high-school graduate, and works in a laundromat. He is "a Christian who tries to live according to the Bible," but is not associated with any particular religious institution. Before contracting genital herpes one month ago, Bruce had no chronic illness or STD, and knew little of the disease.

The herpes outbreak was extremely painful, lasting for 20 days. The primary area of infection was the penis, resulting in difficulty walking due to friction, burning sensations when urinating, and difficulty sleeping. He used medication at the onset of the disease, and avoided liquids. Bruce blames a 24 year old acquaintance of four months for infecting him, although she denies having previous outbreaks. He was "completely surprised" to learn he had herpes since, unlike North Americans, he only has sex the "normal" way (i.e., no oral-genital sex) and he and his partner were both "clean." His anger toward his partner, who he stopped seeing immediately, subsided after a few days, as he realized "it didn't make sense." Other feelings included shock, denial, shame, depression, embarrassment, guilt and self-blame because he had failed to live according to the Bible. He felt life was not worth living, equating the disease with cancer after reading a pamphlet indicating that there is no cure. He considers herpes "dirty and disgusting," feeling God is punishing him for his transgression, but prays for healing. He used to feel obliged to have intercourse daily, because his friend expected it. Due to his fear of transmitting the disease he now has sex with no one, and has been careful not to let friends know that he has herpes. He is sure his Christian friends would reject him, as he would do the same in their place. Bruce's greatest fear is losing his fiancée who he knows he should, in fairness, inform that he has genital herpes. He emphasized that sexual mores are less free in Trinidad, and although he visited his fiancée there, he avoided telling her of his disease. She noticed he shunned physical contact and has become more introspective. If he did not plan to marry, he now thinks he would prefer celibacy.

Professionals contacted have included two doctors and a nurse, all of whom tried to comfort him and assure him that his health was not seriously endangered. Bruce does not feel that a social worker could help him with his very emotional response to herpes. However, he knows he will need to talk to someone about his relationship with his fiancée, which he anticipates will be complicated by his disinterest in sexual activity. Social workers could play a role in informing and reassuring herpes sufferers, but only a cure would be of interest to him.

Case #3 (Recurrent Outbreak)

Cathy is a 28 year old Caucasian English-Canadian working as a doctor's receptionist. She married at age 18, after high school, but is separated and living with her 26 year old partner. She has no children. She believes in God and in the Bible, but was never baptized in the Catholic religion, to which her father belonged. She had never had a chronic illness or STD until just over one year ago, when she had her first genital herpes outbreak, which lasted for two weeks. Symptoms were internal and painful, and included difficulty urinating and a swollen stomach, which made her look pregnant and changed her body image. The only medication used was an ointment given to her as part of the clinic's experimental treatment program during a recurrence. She also took hot baths three or four times daily for pain relief. During her six recurrences, the primary area of infection has been the external genitals, and once, the buttocks. Recurrences cause less discomfort than the first outbreak, unless a new area is infected; she pretends they do not exist, and always hopes each recurrence will be her last.

Cathy and her partner experienced first outbreaks simultaneously, but she believes that she got herpes from a casual relationship, of which her partner is unaware, when on vacation alone. She had little prior knowledge about this disease, but felt she could not get it, since she did not plan to sleep with anyone other than her boyfriend. They were together when diagnosed, and were both shocked, feeling they were given a "death sentence." When her partner then suggested the disease "bound them together for life" she felt trapped, but would fear transmitting herpes to a new partner, who she would have to tell she has herpes. Feelings experienced upon learning she was afflicted included a sense of unreality, depression, and dirtiness. She "felt like killing the guy" who infected her, but generalized negative feelings to all men. She also felt guilty and angry with herself for infecting her partner. Cathy feels God is punishing her for leaving her husband, having a casual affair, and being a carrier. She feels "unworthy" to be in the company of her family and that of her boyfriend, and has only confided in a close friend. Before contracting herpes she felt that having sex about once a week was a necessary, pleasurable, and exciting part of her relationship. She now has sex only once a month, but recognizes that this is due, in part, to a deteriorating relationship quite apart from the disease. Still, herpes has decreased her pleasure and made her less spontaneous, fearing a recurrence will be triggered. She and her partner no longer engage in oral-genital sex.

The nurse, who she found warm and helpful, and a doctor, who was very "technical" in orientation were the only professionals seen regarding herpes. Although wondering how others cope, Cathy declined an offer of group therapy, fearing she might meet someone she knows. She was unaware of self-help groups. Cathy never told the psychologist she is seeing for "emotional problems" that she has genital herpes. She feels that a social worker could help sufferers by providing up-to-date information, lending support, and building confidence when a person enters a new relationship, especially by helping them handle ethical issues related to their condition.

Case #4 (Recurrence)

Don is a 25 year old Caucasian, born in Italy, who has lived in Canada since the age of two years. He is single and lives with his parents. He has been dating someone for six months. Following high school, he took a hairdressing course, and is employed in a beauty salon. He considers himself "somewhat religious," meaning that he observes Catholic holidays. Before contracting genital herpes one and one-half years ago, Don had never had a chronic illness or STD. He acquired herpes from a women he was dating at the time. His first outbreak was not physically painful. The primary area of infection was under the foreskin of his penis. The four recurrences, which have been less discomforting, have been in the same area as the first outbreak, and are not always visible.

Don was poorly informed about genital herpes before getting it, but knew that cold sores "were not fatal." He was "completely surprised" to find that he had herpes and never thought he would be "one of those people" who got an STD. He blamed and resented his former partner, who he feels had not been totally honest when saying she did not know she had herpes. He suspected she had been seeing another man, and stopped dating her, or anyone, for three months. He also blamed himself for not being "more selective." Other feelings included depression, loneliness, and a fear of rejection. He wondered if he would be able to lead a normal life and have children. He coped with his immediate feelings by taking a few days off to pull himself "together" and obtain information about genital herpes. His loneliness decreased gradually, as he was finally able to confide in close friends, whom he found understanding and supportive, although surprised that someone like him had this disease. Before having herpes, Don had sex about three times a week and found it enjoyable. Now, he no longer engages in sexual activity as early in relationships as he did before. Also, he distances himself from his partners during recurrences, which he compared to women having to "abstain" during menstruation. The person he is seeing now knows that he has herpes and is understanding. Other than an ointment the clinic provided as part of an experimental treatment, Don has used no medication. However, he believes stress, fatigue, and overwork, trigger recurrences, and tries to rest and use relaxation techniques when they occur. He feels he has learned to cope with the disease well on his own.

Don only saw a nurse whom he found extremely helpful, suggesting that one could live a normal life with herpes. He has never participated in any type of therapy, did not know of self-help groups previously, and does not feel they would help him. He does think a social worker should be able to help a person coping with genital herpes by answering questions, offering guidance, and being an understanding and good listener.

SUMMARY AND RECOMMENDATIONS

The above cases are illustrative of many of the psychosocial aspects of genital herpes that are often overlooked when emphasis is placed mainly on the medical aspects of the disease. Although medical symptoms follow the predictable, if variable, pattern suggested in the literature, the complexity of individual, interpersonal, and sociocultural variables involved may cause psychosocial responses to be more difficult to predict. The influence of cultural factors was clearly evident in these volunteers, who happened to represent four different cultural backgrounds. Despite the fact that all of them reside in the same city and have been exposed to the same media coverage about herpes, their idiosyncratic responses must be viewed in the light of additional sociocultural factors such as prior knowledge of the disease, place of birth, ethnic background, and religious beliefs (Christensen, 1983). Cultural factors also played a significant role in determining the degree of psychological and interpersonal stress engendered by the diagnosis. Self-esteem was most severely damaged, and the emotional scars deepest, in the two cases where the disease was seen as "punishment," and hurtful to loved ones. Several recognizable stages in the natural adjustment process (Luby and Gillespie, 1981) were experienced, and the need for support and reassurance was clearly indicated. All four respondents could envision a role for the social worker in relieving the psychosocial effects of the disease.

In summary, it is recommended that social workers resolve to take a more active role in treating psychosocial aspects of genital herpes, which could involve some or all of the following activities:

1. Provision of accurate and up-to-date information, and referral to medical, psychotherapeutic, and self-help sources.
2. Providing victims opportunities for ventilation and clarification of feelings in a non-judgmental atmosphere as an adjunct to other services in medical, school, and community settings.
3. Using counselling skills and conjoint interviewing techniques, to help individuals, couples, and groups to deal with ethical issues relating to genital herpes.
4. Participating in public awareness campaigns and efforts to change agency policies in order to allow those afflicted with herpes and other STDs more ready access to the services of professionals and self-help groups.

Depending on the setting, opportunities for the use of various skills and techniques will be presented to the worker willing to offer help to herpes victims. As front line workers, policy-makers, and researchers, social workers are in an excellent position to play a leading role in responding to the psychosocial aspects of genital herpes.

REFERENCES

Bettoli, E.J. (1982). Herpes: Facts and fallacies. *American Journal of Nursing*, June, 924-929.

Christensen, C.P. (1983). The influence of culture in undergraduate sexuality education: A course experience. *Intervention, 65-66*, Fall/Winter, 58-63.

Cuthbert, M. (1981). Herpes: Towards a positive approach. *Healthsharing*, Winter, 15-18.

Drob, S. (1984, August). *Psychotherapy with patients suffering from genital herpes*. Presented at 92nd Annual Convention of the American Psychological Association, Toronto, 1-17.

Drob, S. & Bernard, H.S. (1986). Time-limited group treatment of genital herpes patients. *International Journal of Group Psychotherapy, 36*(1), 133-144.

Gallagher, N. (1982). Fever all through the night. *Mother Jones, VII* (IX), 36-43.

Gillespie, O. (1982). *Herpes: What to do when you have it*. New York: Grosset & Dunlap Inc.

Greenwood, V.B. & Bernstein, R.A. (1982). *Coping with herpes: The emotional problems*. Washington, D.C.: The Washington Center for Cognitive-Behavioural Therapy.

Gulas, I. & Griffiths, L. (1984). *Herpes: The love bug, facts and fears*. Columbus, Ohio: Ohio Psychology Publishing Co.

Hamilton, R. (1980). *The herpes book*. Los Angeles: J. P. Tarcher Inc.

Lawee, D. (1982). Genital herpetic infection: A family practice perspective. *Canadian Family Physician, 28,* 1839-1848.

Luby, E. & Gillespie, O. (1981). Psychological responses to genital herpes. *The Helper, 3*(4), 2-3.

Manne, S., Sandler, I., & Zautra, A. (1986). Coping and adjustment to genital herpes: The effects of time and social support. *Journal of Behavioral Medicine, 9*(2), 163-177.

Montreal Health Press Inc. (1984). *A book about sexually transmitted diseases*.

Reichman, R.C., Badger, G.J., Mertz, G.J. et al. (1984). Treatment of recurrent genital herpes simplex infections with oral acyclovir. A controlled trial. *Journal of the American Medical Association, 251,* 2103-2107.

Sacks, S.L. (1983). *The truth about herpes*. Toronto/Montreal, Grosvenor House Press, Inc.

Woodis, C. (1983). Herpes genitalis: The benefits of self-help groups for sufferers. *The Practitioner, 227*(1379), 865-866.

AIDS and Social Work: Sociopsychological Training Curriculum for Human Sexuality and Related Fields of Professional Practice

Steven P. Schinke
Robert F. Schilling
Marian S. Krauskopf
Gilbert J. Botvin
Mario A. Orlandi

INTRODUCTION

Social workers in practice and research on human sexuality are well acquainted with the magnitude and consequences of Acquired Immune Deficiency Syndrome (AIDS). As social workers in New York City, the authors are acutely aware of the prevalence, incidence, and effects of AIDS. Home to the bulk of the country's diagnosed AIDS and AIDS-related complex (ARC) cases, New York City also has the nation's largest concentrations of high-risk groups for human immunodeficiency virus (HIV) infection associated with AIDS and ARC. These high-risk groups are intravenous drug users, homosexual men, heterosexual women and men with

© 1988 by The Haworth Press, Inc. All rights reserved.

bisexual partners, and women of childbearing age who inject drugs or who are prostitutes (Deuchar, 1984; Perry & Tross, 1984). As such, New York City reports a higher prevalence of and incidence for heterosexual transmission of HIV than any other U.S. city.

Based on our clinical and research experience in New York City and on the scientific literature, in the following three sections we describe curricula for training social workers to effectively and ethically serve persons with or at risk for AIDS and ARC. In the first section we briefly outline a format and theoretical rationale for in-service training on AIDS intended for social workers in human sexuality and other practice settings. Next, in the second section we detail essential curriculum elements for that training. The third section gives an evaluation scheme for documenting the outcomes and impact of professional training for social work practice around AIDS issues. The paper concludes with an agenda for future social work practice and research in human sexuality and other fields related to AIDS, ARC, and HIV infection.

AIDS EDUCATION CURRICULA

Format and Theory

Training for social work practitioners to deal with sexual and sociopsychological aspects of HIV infection, ARC, and AIDS will necessarily occur within in-service or continuing education formats. Whatever the context, training delivery would ideally follow a sequence of initial didactic instruction, small group experiential procedures, and subsequent booster, or updating sessions. Required by virtue of emerging scientific and practice knowledge on AIDS, ARC, and HIV, booster sessions could be ongoing, every 4 to 6 months after initial instruction. In human sexuality areas, if not in other fields of profession practice, training leaders ought to represent an interdisciplinary approach to AIDS.

Elsewhere, for example, the authors have suggested the advantages of interdisciplinary teams of social workers, nurses, immunologists, psychiatrists, and such members of interested constituencies as gay health care, counselling, and lay community representatives, union officials, hospital administrators, and representatives from the corporate and private sectors (Feldman, 1986). Besides their complementary substantive expertise, these interdisciplinary teams and members can bring variety and interest to training, thereby enhancing the attraction and attendance of social work practitioner participants.

To understand human sexuality and sociopsychological issues regarding AIDS and ARC, social work practitioners need a theoretical and empirical grounding in salient, state-of-the-art information. Theoretical guidance for social work practice in this area can benefit from an ecological, systems-approach perspective (cf. Akabas & Kurzman, 1982; Germain & Gitterman, 1980; Meyer, 1983; Whittaker, Schinke, & Gilchrist, in press). This perspective can inform not only AIDS curricula content, but also the processes through which the curricula are delivered. For instance, curricula on medical, psychiatric, and sociobehavioral issues of AIDS and ARC can help social workers understand and positively influence the interactive forces between person, or individual, variables and environment variables on clients and on clients' families and employers.

Curricula Elements

To integrate the latest scientific and clinical knowledge, training curricula for social work practice can profit from an emerging body of published literature on AIDS, ARC, and HIV infection (Altman, 1986; Batchelor, 1984; Bloom, Abrams, & Rodgers, 1986; Douglas & Kallam, 1985; Lusby, 1985; Nichols, 1985; Nichols & Ostrow, 1984; Nurnberg, Prudic, Fiori et al., 1984; Simmons-Alling, 1984; Smith & Ryan, 1984; Wachter, 1986; Weibe, 1986). Training curricula can begin with data on the nature, etiology, diagnosis, correlates, and consequences of HIV infection (Centers for Disease Control, 1986; Curran et al., 1985; Mass, 1985; McKusick, Horstman, & Coates, 1985; Siegal & Siegal, 1983; Weiss, Saxinger, Rechtman et al., 1985). Other content should acquaint practitioners with differences between AIDS and ARC (Morin, Charles, & Malyon, 1984). Specific attention should focus on psychiatric and sociopsychological complications, ethics, family issues, children, ethnic-racial minority group members, intravenous drug users, heterosexual at risk groups, prevention, and workplace issues.

Psychiatric and sociopsychological complications of AIDS and ARC encompass a host of issues (Coates, Temoshok, & Mandel, 1984; Kinnier, 1986; Korcok, 1985). These include psychoneuroimmunology, or the confluence of stress and coping variables that may partially modulate immunity and immunologically resisted diseases (cf. Jemmot & Locke, 1984; Solomon, in press). Also covered in this content should be issues of depression, anxiety, stress reaction, hypochondria, and obsessive ruminations among AIDS and ARC patients (Ferrara, 1984; Landesman, Ginzburg, & Weiss, 1985; Quinn, 1985). Also, practitioners should be acquainted with differing psychiatric and sociopsychological needs of AIDS victims, ARC clients, and those who manifest no evidence of AIDS or ARC, but are no less anxious — the so-called "worried well" (Holland & Tross, 1985; Joseph, Emmons, Kessler et al., 1984). Social workers should also learn about such techniques for dealing with these groups as positive coping behaviors, cognitive restructuring procedures, and social and informal support networks (Miller & Green, 1985).

Workers should learn about stresses experienced by ARC patients and about how these patients can cope with their diagnosis (Korcok, 1985). Likewise, workers can grow familiar with the needs of high-risk persons who, though not diagnosed as AIDS or ARC patients, are nonetheless concerned over their future health and well-being. Insurance coverage issues — including health and life insurance — should also be discussed in professional education for social work with AIDS clients. Specific attention should be given to the problems and needs of patients, family, significant others, employers, coworkers, and insurers in providing health and life coverage for AIDS, ARC, and HIV patients and higher risk groups (cf. Akabas, 1984).

In addition, training for social workers in human sexuality and other fields of practice should show how stress and anxiety may further exacerbate immunosuppression and increase risk of acquiring AIDS (Dilley, Ochitill, Perl et al., 1985). Similarly, trainees should be acquainted with the possible interactions between emotional states and disease severity among AIDS and ARC clients. Workers should be acquainted with neuropathological consequences of HIV, including memory loss, depression, and other signs of dementia. Practitioners should at least learn clues to help them distinguish between characteristics of dementia, emotional problems, and drug side effects among HIV seropositive patients. Furthermore, workers ought to be familiarized with the probable interactive influences of genetic, environmental, lifestyle, substance use, and affective variables on an individual's risk for and response to AIDS.

Ethical content for social work with HIV, ARC, and AIDS patients should emphasize methods for informing patients of seropositive HIV results. Other topics for inclusion in ethical content are cost-effective issues around providing expensive medical treatment to AIDS patients, decisions about the time to discharge AIDS patients from hospitals, and the clinical impact of philosophical discussions surrounding definitions of humane treatment for AIDS clients (Skeen, 1985; Steinbrook, Lo, Moulton, et al., 1985). Ethics content should further address legal issues related to AIDS, ARC, and HIV infected patients.

Family related content should help workers recognize the burdens of those who may concurrently learn that someone has AIDS and is gay, bisexual, or an intravenous drug user. Among practitioners, this content can sharpen trainees' skill with family counseling issues. Specifically, workers can learn to help family members recognize early signs of neuropathology, including memory loss, impaired concentration, and severe depression. Social workers should additionally receive guidelines for advising family members about seeking neuropsychiatric consultation to differentiate problems of dementia from drug side effects, anxieties, and emotional disorders. Last, workers can be acquainted with procedures for family members, friends, and significant others to assist AIDS and ARC clients with everyday tasks and routines.

Children with or at risk for HIV infection should also be discussed in training for social workers. Here, training should focus on diagnostic, treatment, ethical, and prevention concerns. Recommendations from the Centers for Disease Control regarding school attendance, day care participation, and peer group contact among children with AIDS ought to be presented and discussed (Boland & Gaskill, 1984; Nichols, 1983; Price, 1986; Price, Navia, & Cho, 1986; Reed, 1986).

Ethnic-racial minority group content should acquaint social workers with HIV infection incidence and prevalence data on Black, Haitian, Puerto Rican, Colombian, Cuban and Dominican Americans (Morgan, Curran, 1986). For example, Table 1 shows current and projected AIDS cases for American adults divided by the three major ethnic-racial groups. Consequently, workers must learn why clinicians and researchers must carefully distinguish among and within ethnic-racial minority groups relative to HIV, ARC, and AIDS risks and treatment strategies (Schinke, Schilling, & Gilchrist, in press). Recent data, in fact, project ascending rates of HIV infection among majority culture populations relative to ethnic racial minority groups (Morgen & Curren, 1986).

Intravenous drug users, due to the risk of AIDS in this group, warrant special attention. To a greater degree than homosexual or bisexual men, intravenous drug users are stigmatized in America (Jonsen, Cooke, & Koenig, 1986). An unfortunate outcome of this stigma is that drug users with AIDS and ARC are apt to receive little professional attention. In New York City, nearly one-third of all AIDS victims are intravenous drug users. Workers should know that intravenous drug users face two major risks for HIV infection. First, habitual users of injected drugs have weakened immune systems. Second, their sharing of unsterile needles increases users' exposure to HIV (Pincus, 1984). Given these circumstances, workers must learn tactics for effectively working with intravenous drug users so that each problem area – drug use and AIDS – is handled responsibly. Toward this end, workers should learn that among New York City intravenous drug users, nearly 60% are willing to change their drug taking habits – including stopping drug use, not sharing needles, and using sterile needles (Drug Use and AIDS, 1986).

Heterosexual at-risk groups also have salience for social workers in human sexuality. Thus, workers can learn that nearly one-half of American women with AIDS live in New York City and that one in seven of these women got HIV through heterosexual contacts. This material can lead to presentations of risk factors for heterosexual

Table 1

Recorded and Projected AIDS Cases for American Adults

	Recorded			Projected	
	1983	1984	1985	1986	1991
Hispanic	586	747	1,227	2,300	10,800
Black	1,036	1,307	2,114	3,700	15,200
White	2,294	3,270	5,256	9,500	46,900
Other	69	59	81	100	100
Total	3,967	5,383	8,678	15,600	73,000

Note: From "Acquired Immunodeficiency Syndrome: Current and Future Trends" by W.M. Morgan and J.W. Curran, 1986, *Public Health Reports: Journal of the U.S. Public Health Service*, *101*, p. 463. No copyright held; U.S. government material in the public domain.

women and men relative to such variables as bisexuality, drug use, prostitution, and sexual practices. Particular attention should be given to commonalities and differences among risk factors for HIV infection relative to heterosexual issues (cf. Cohen & Weisman, 1986). Training here can focus on procedures for screening heterosexual populations for AIDS, ethical considerations when tests reveal HIV positive results, and preventive intervention strategies (Eckholm, 1985; McKusick, Wiley, Coates, et al., 1985). Last, similar and differential HIV risk reduction strategies for women and for men should be discussed (Acquired Immune Deficiency Syndrome, 1982; Recommendations for Prevention, 1986).

Prevention content aimed at HIV transmission, ARC, and AIDS should be introduced through the available scientific and clinical evidence to support effective strategies (Potter & Pritchard, 1986).

Practitioners should review prevention methods that account for lifestyle, personal choice, and sociobehavioral variables around HIV transmission risk. Preventive methods aimed at the individual and at the larger environment can also be detailed. For instance, data on individual strategies for preventing AIDS and for increasing cellular immunity could be reviewed (Kiecolt-Glaser, Glaser, Strain, et al., 1986). Environmental strategies at community, government, and policy making levels can similarly be presented (Burda & Powills, 1986; Devita, Hellman, & Rosenberg, 1983; Mills, Wofsy, & Mills, 1986; Nichols, 1986). For instance, workers should be aware of the relative costs and benefits of mass media, educational, and individually based approaches to AIDS prevention.

Workplace issues for professional training can address the needs of those who interact with AIDS and ARC clients by vocation (e.g., health care providers) and those who work with such clients by circumstance (co-workers of these clients). Curricula related to both levels of concern should discuss the risks of HIV transmission through causal or accidental contacts. Likewise, the psychological stresses and tensions of working closely with AIDS and ARC patients should be covered. Workers who serve AIDS populations should additionally discuss such issues as emotional attachment to clients, pressures from too heavy a caseload, and bereavement (Dunkel & Hatfield, 1986; Furstenberg & Olson, 1984; Lee, 1986; Lopez & Getzel, 1984). For this content, workers should meet in small groups to facilitate candid, open discussions about personal and professional concerns.

Material related to workplace issues should be included to help social work practitioners learn how to effectively counsel people who, as co-workers, have regular contact with HIV patients (Akabas, 1984; Busto, 1986; Lambda Legal Defense and Education, 1984; National Association of Social Workers, 1984). Such counseling can have two objectives. First, practitioners can learn to reduce fears among co-wokers about their being infected with HIV from AIDS and ARC patients. Second, practitioners can learn strategies to enhance co-workers' support, communications, and stress reduction efforts with AIDS and ARC victims.

Admmittedly brief, this outline of curricula for training social workers in human sexuality and other settings to work effectively with issues surrounding AIDS suggests the breadth and depth of material essential to professional services.

EVALUATION

Because professional training is effective only if it leads to behavior change, the effects of AIDS and ARC curricula must be evaluated. One pragmatic and ethically sound evaluation method is a pretest, posttest, and follow-up research design. With this design, each social worker participant is pretested prior to training. Pretests can measure workers' knowledge of AIDS, ARC, and HIV. Attitudinal measures can ask workers about their current or future interactions with such AIDS subgroups as children, ethnic-racial minority persons, heterosexual at risk groups, and intravenous drug users. Other measures could document workers' perceived clinical skills with AIDS, ARC, and HIV infected clients.

Clinical skills questions could measure workers' ability to conduct client assessments, to identify neuropsychiatric, behavioral, psychological, and physical signs of early and advanced AIDS and ARC, to design treatment and intervention strategies, to suggest preventive interventions for limiting HIV transmission, and to involve family members and significant others in treatment and prevention efforts around AIDS, ARC, and HIV. A final schedule of questions could ask workers to estimate their comfort, anxiety, and preferences for working with various groups of HIV patients.

Social work training participants could then be retested at the end of curricula delivery and 6 months later. Posttest and 6-month follow-up measures could be similar to pretest measures, with items and scales reordered to reduce response biases. At posttest and at a 6-month follow-up after curricular delivery, quality of care measures could also be completed by AIDS, ARC, HIV seropositive, or high-risk clients seen by training participants. After giving their informed consent, selected clients could be given questionnaires about the nature, quality, and efficacy of services they received from the index workers.

To be sure, pretest to post-test and follow-up improvement among social workers could result from influences extraneous to training. But the feasibility of a before and after design, together with multiple data sources, affords a practical evaluation strategy that can yield empirical support for the impact and benefits of professional training on AIDS, ARC, and HIV.

CONCLUSIONS

AIDS is a problem that social workers in human sexuality practice and research cannot ignore. Without question, as shown earlier in Table 1, the magnitude and effects of AIDS, ARC, and HIV infection will grow more pervasive in social work practice before they diminish. According to the Centers for Disease Control:

> AIDS will become an even more serious public health problem in the United States during the next 5 years with a concurrent need for medical and social services for AIDS patients. . . . Our current understanding of the severity of AIDS and projections for the future underscore the need for continued commitment to research for a vaccine and therapy. Primary prevention and education activities must be widely implemented now throughout the United States to curtail the further spread of infection and future AIDS cases. (Morgan & Curran, 1986, p. 464)

Until such treatment and preventive interventions are available and effective, social work practitioners must deal with myriad, complex, and unprecedented tasks around service provision to AIDS clients, their families and significant others, and their employers.

Quality, state-of-the-art professional training to educate social workers about AIDS and related issues its timely and needed. This paper is a modest step toward that training. Drawn from the scientific literature and from our clinical and research experience in the U.S. city most affected by AIDS, the curricula and guidelines offered here provide a beginning for professional social work in-service training. The described curricula could provide a foundation for more efforts to educate professionals about AIDS, ARC, and

HIV. We urge our colleagues to build, refine, and improve the curricula and directions for its use within and outside the social work community.

In the process of describing our curricula, implementation format, and evaluation scheme, we found several issues that warrant future attention. Among the most pressing of these issues is the need for innovative vehicles for educating social workers about AIDS. Doubtless, the scholarly literature such as the present publication is the most respected and recognized vehicle for such dissemination. To date, however, the bulk of the literature on AIDS has not come from social work or from kindred human services professions and has not been aimed at our clinical interests. More forums such as this journal therefore need to help educate our colleagues.

New and carefully controlled research by social workers can enhance the scientific knowledge base and the level of agency and clinical services relative to AIDS, ARC, and HIV. Social workers in the human sexuality field and in other fields of practice are increasingly demonstrating their expertise as clinical researchers. The available research capacity and creativity ought to be applied in the service of helping the profession to better serve persons with and at risk for AIDS.

REFERENCES

Acquired Immune Deficiency Syndrome (AIDS): Precautions for Clinical and Laboratory Staffs (1982). *Morbidity and mortality weekly report, 31,* 577-580.

Akabas, S.H. (1984). Expanded view for worksite counselor. *Business and Health,* December, pp. 24-28.

Akabas, S.H. & Kurzman, P.A. (1982). The industrial social welfare specialist: What's so special. In S.H. Akabas & P.A. Kurzman (Eds.), *Work, workers and work organizations,* (pp. 197-235). Englewood Cliffs, NJ: Prentice-Hall.

Altman, D. (1986). *AIDS in the mid of America.* New York: Doubleday.

Batchelor, W.F. (1984). AIDS: A public health and psychological emergency. *American Psychologist, 39,* 1279-1284.

Bloom, E.J., Abrams, D.T., & Rogers, G.R. (1986). Lupus anticoagulant in the acquired immunodeficiency syndrome. *The Journal of the American Medical Association, 256,* 491-493.

Boland, M., & Gaskill, T.D. (1984). Managing AIDS in children. *American Journal of Maternal and Child Nursing, 9,* 384-389.

Burda, D., & Powills, S. (1986). AIDS: A time bomb at hospitals' door. *Hospitals, 60,* 54-61.

Busto, M.R. (1986). AIDS in the work place. *The Bar Bulletin.*

Centres for Disease Control. (1986). *Reports on AIDS published in the morbidity and mortality weekly report, June 1981 through February 1986.* Springfield, VA: National Technical Information Service.

Coates, T.J., Temshok, L., & Mandel, J. (1984). Psychosocial research is essential to understanding and treating AIDS. *American Psychologist, 39,* 1309-1314.

Cohen, M.A. & Weisman, H.W. (1986). A biopsychosocial approach to AIDS. *Psychosomatics, 27,* 245-249.

Curran, J.W., & Morgan, W.M. (1986). Acquired immunodeficiency syndrome: Current and future trends. *Public Health Reports: Journal of the U.S. Public Health Service, 101,* 459-465.

Curran, J.W., Morgan, W.M., Hardy, A.M., et al. (1985). The epidemiology of AIDS: Current status and future prospects. *Science, 229,* 1352-1357.

Deuchar, N. (1984). AIDS in New York City with particular reference to the psycho-social aspects. *British Journal of Psychiatry, 145,* 612-619.

Devita, V., Hellman, S., & Rosenberg, S. (1985). *AIDS: Etiology, diagnosis, treatment, and prevention.* New York: Lippincott.

Dilley, J.W., Ochitill, H.N., Perl, M., et al. (1985). Findings in psychiatric consultations with patients with acquired immune deficiency syndrome. *American Journal of Psychiatry, 142,* 82-86.

Douglas, C.J., & Kalam, T. (1985). Homophobia among physicians and nurses: An empirical study. *Hospital and Community Psychiatry, 36,* 1309-1311.

Drug Use and AIDS (1986). *Alcohol, drug abuse, and mental health news. 12*(5), 1; 8.

Dunkel, J., & Hatfield, S. (1986). Countertransference issues in working with persons with AIDS. *Social Work, 31,* 114-118.

Eckholm, E. (1985). Women and AIDS: Assessing the risks. *New York Times,* October 28, 1985, C-1.

Feldman, R.A. (1986). Training for health care providers to address acquired immune deficiency syndrome (AIDS). Grant proposal submitted to National Institute of Mental Health by Columbia University School of Social Work, New York, NY.

Ferrara, A.J. (1984). My personal experience with AIDS. *American Psychologist, 39,* 1285-1287.

Furstenberg, A., & Olson, M.M. (1984). Social work and AIDS. *Social Work in Health Care, 9,* 45-62.

Germain, C.B., & Gitterman, A. (1980). *The life model of social work practice.* New York: Columbia University Press.

Holland, J.C., & Tross, S. (1985). The psychological and neuropsychiatric sequelae of the acquired immunodeficiency syndrome and related disorders. *Annals of Internal Medicine, 103,* 760-764.

Jemmot, J.B., & Locke, S.E. (1984). Psychosocial factors, immunological mediation, and human susceptibility to infectious diseases. *Psychological Bulletin, 95,* 78-108.

Jonsen, A.R., Cooke, M., & Koenig, B.A. (1986). AIDS and ethics. *Issues in Science and Technology, 2,* 56-65.

Joseph, J.G., Emmons, C.A., Kessler, R.C., et al. (1984). Coping with the threat of AIDS: An approach to sociopsychological assessment. *American Psychologist, 39,* 1297-1302.

Kiecolt-Glaser, J.K., Glaser, R., Strain, E.C., et al. (1986). Modulation of cellular immunity in medical students. *Journal of Behavioral Medicine, 9,* 5-21.

Kinnier, R.T. (1986). The need for sociopsychological research on AIDS and counselling interventions for AIDS victims. *Journal of Counseling and Development, 64,* 472-474.

Korcok, M. (1985). AIDS hysteria: A contagious side effect *Canadian Medical Association Journal, 133,* 1241-1248.

Lambda Legal Defense and Education Fund (1984). *AIDS legal guide: A professional resource on AIDS-related legal issues and discrimination.* New York: Author.

Landesman, S.H., Ginzburg, H.M., & Weiss, S.H. (1985). The AIDS epidemic. *New England Journal of Medicine, 312,* 521-525.

Lee, P.R. (1986). AIDS: Allocating resources for research and patient care. *Issues in Science and Technology, 2,* 66-73.

Lopez, D.J., & Getzel, G.S. (1984). Helping gay AIDS patients in crisis. *Social Casework, 65,* 387-394.

Lusby, G. (1985). AIDS: The impact on the health care worker. *Frontiers of Radiation Therapy and Oncology, 19,* 164-167.

Mass, L. (1985). *Medical answers about AIDS.* New York: Gay Men's Health Crisis.

McKusick, L., Horstman, W., & Coates, T.J. (1985). AIDS and sexual behavior reported by gay men in San Francisco. *American Journal of Public Health. 75,* 493-496.

McKusick, L., Wiley, J.A., Coates, T.J. , et al. (1985). Reported changes in the sexual behavior of men at risk for AIDS, San Francisco, 1982-84: The AIDS behavioral research project. *Public Health Reports, 100,* 622-629.

Meyer, C.H. (1983). The search for coherence. In C.H. Meyer (ed.), *Clinical social work in the eco-systems perspective* (pp. 5-34). New York: Columbia University Press.

Mills, M., Wofsy, C.B., & Mills, J. (1986). The acquired immunodeficiency syndrome: Infection control and public health law. *New England Journal of Medicine, 314,* 457-460.

Miller, D., & Green, J. (1985). Psychological support and counselling for patients with acquired immune deficiency syndrome (AIDS). *Genitourinary Medicine, 61,* 273-278.

Morin, S.F., Charles, K.A., & Malyon, A. K. (1984). The psychological impact of AIDS on gay men. *American Psychologist, 39,* 1288-1293.

Morgan, W.M., & Curran, J.W. (1986). Acquired immunodeficiency syndrome: Current and future trends. *Public Health Reports: Journal of the U.S. Public Health Service, 101,* 459-465.

National Association of Social Workers. (1984). *Acquired immune deficiency syndrome (AIDS): A policy statement.* Silver Spring, MD: Author.

Nichols, E.K. (1986). *Mobilizing against AIDS: The unfinished story of a virus.* Cambridge: Harvard University Press.

Nichols, S.E. (1983). Psychiatric aspects of AIDS. *Psychsomatics, 24,* 1083-1089.

Nichols, S.E. (1985). Psychosocial reactions of persons with acquired immunodeficiency syndrome. *Annals of Internal Medicine, 103,* 765-767.

Nichols, S.E., & Ostrow, D.G. (1984). *Psychiatric implications of the acquired immune deficiency syndrome.* Washington, DC: American Psychiatric Press.

Nurnberg, H.G., Prudic, J., Fiori, M., et al. (1984). Psychopathology complicating acquired immune deficiency syndrome (AIDS). *American Journal of Psychiatry, 141,* 95-96.

Perry, S.W., & Tross, S. (1984). Psychiatric problems of AIDS inpatients at the New York Hospital: Preliminary report. *Public Health Reports, 99,* 200-205.

Pincus, H.A. (1984). AIDS, drug abuse, and mental health. *Public Health Reports, 99,* 106-108.

Potter, G.C., & Pritchard, R.E. (1986). *Preventing AIDS: Facts and myths.* Wenonah, NJ: University Information Associates.

Price, J.H. (1986). AIDS, the schools, and policy issues. *Journal of School Health, 56,* 137-140.

Price, R.W., Navia, B.A., & Cho, E.S. (1986). AIDS encephalopathy. *Neurologic Clinics, 4,* 285-301.

Quinn, T.L. (1985). Perspectives on the future of AIDS. *Journal of the American Medical Association, 253,* 247-249.

Recommendations for Preventing Transmission of Infection with Human T. Lymphotropic Virus Type III/Lymphadenopathy-Associated Virus during Invasive Procedures. (1986). *Morbidity and mortality weekly report, 35,* 221-223.

Reed, S. (1986). AIDS in the schools: A special report. *Phi Delta Kappa,* March, *44,* 494-498.

Schinke, S.P., Schilling, R.F., & Gilchrist, L.D. (in press). Hispanic and Black adolescents, prevention, and health promotion. *Behavioral Medicine Abstracts.*

Siegal, F.P., & Siegal, M.S. (1983). *AIDS: The medical mystery.* New York: Grove Press.

Simmons-Alling, S. (1984). AIDS: Psychosocial needs of the health care worker. *Topics in Clinical Nursing, 6,* 31-37.

Smith, D., & Ryan, C.C. (1984). Psychosocial issues for people with AIDS. *Journal of Medical Association of Georgia, 73,* 535-536.

Solomon, G.F. (in press). The emerging field of psychoneuroimmunology. *Journal of Psychosomatic Research.*

Skeen, W.F. (1985). Acquired immunodeficiency syndrome and the emergency physician. *Annals of Emergency Medicine, 14,* 267-273.

Steinbrook, R., Lo, B. , & Moulton, J., et al. (1985). Ethical dilemmas in caring for patients with the acquired immunodeficiency syndrome. *Annals of Internal Medicine, 103,* 787-980.

Wachter, R.M. (1986). The impact of the acquired immunodeficiency syndrome on medical residency training. *New England Journal of Medicine, 314,* 177-186.

Weibe, C. (1986). Professional demands, human frailties: Doctors respond to AIDS. *New Physician, 35,* 14-36.

Weiss, S.H., Saxinger, W.C., Rechtman, D., et al. (1985). HIV infection among health care workers. *Journal of the American Medical Association,* 254, 2089-2093.

Whittaker, J. K., Schinke, S.P., & Gilchrist, L.D. (in press). Ecological approaches to skills training and social network interventions. *Social Service Review.*

Learning About the Psychosocial Impact of Sexually Transmitted Diseases: Teaching Strategies

John R. Moore

INTRODUCTION

Education about sexually transmitted diseases (STD) primarily has been focused on its medical aspects. Textbooks and other instructional materials present information on etiologic agents, symptoms, diagnostic tests, treatments, and complications and sequelae; information that lends itself well to lectures, charts, diagrams, memorization, and testing. However, it is the psychosocial impact of STDs which often has the greatest and longest lasting effect on those people who have STDs (Masters, Johnson, & Kolodny, 1986).

With the major exceptions of herpes and Acquired Immune Deficiency Syndrome (AIDS), most STDs are curable. Prompt detection and treatment minimizes any physical risk and long-term physical problems or complications are not likely. If the STD causes pain or discomfort, the person may limit sexual or other activities during the period of acute symptoms. Many people who become infected have no symptoms or symptoms which are not severe enough to interfere with activity. However, these people might experience feelings of guilt, shame, and embarrassment as a result of being told that they have an STD (Masters, Johnson, & Kolodny, 1986). Drob (1986) found that a diagnosis of herpes could lead to "depression, anxiety, guilt, anger, (and) shame" (p. 100). For some people the psychological reaction can interfere with sexual functioning. These

© 1988 by The Haworth Press, Inc. All rights reserved. *121*

people may feel "contaminated, ugly, damaged, and inferior" (Drob, p. 100). For others the feelings of depression can be severe enough to include suicidal ideation.

The widespread anxiety over AIDS indicates that the psychosocial impact of this sexually transmitted disease affects many more people than just those diagnosed as having AIDS. Understandably, persons with AIDS (PWA) reactions to their condition include:

> Fear of death and dying, guilt, fear of exposure of lifestyle, fear of contagion, loss of self-esteem, fear of loss of physical attractiveness, fears of decreased social support and increased dependency, isolation and stigmatization, loss of occupational and financial status, concerns and confusion over options for medical treatment, and the overriding sense of gloom and helplessness associated with a degenerative illness. (Morin, Charles, & Malyon, 1984, p. 1288)

The stresses associated with a diagnosis of AIDS also can extend to family members and significant others (*Confronting AIDS*, 1986).

Persons who have AIDS Related Complex (ARC) or who have no symptoms but test positive for antibodies to the Human Immunodeficiency Virus (HIV) also experience stress. For these people the future is uncertain. This sense of uncertainty and the presence of ever changing symptoms can result in:

> Intense isolation, reactions to constant reminders of their condition, poor social and occupational functioning due to fatigue, loss of initiative, and frustration of achievement and productivity needs. (Morin, Charles, & Malyon, 1984, p. 1290)

The anxiety associated with AIDS also affects many people who have no symptoms and who do not test positive for HIV antibody (Morin & Batchelor, 1984). Some of these people are members of high risk groups who may or may not have been engaging in high risk behaviors. Others are people who are not members of high risk populations and have not engaged in high risk behaviors but who have been caught up in the general anxiety related to the existence of a fatal illness for which there is no known cure. Adding to this level of anxiety is the amount of AIDS misinformation being spread by media, special interest groups, and even some health professionals.

The emotional trauma which accompanies STD is primarily a function of society's stigmatization of these conditions (Brandt, 1985). In a sex-negative society, a diagnosis of an STD is equated with being immoral and untouchable. We are not able to bring ourselves to talk about STD with the same openness with which we talk about the flu. Although STD and the flu are caused by infectious agents, the implied sexual behavior related to STD prevents us from being comfortable in talking about them. Attribution of blame also plays a role in determining our reactions to diseases. We are "helpless" against flu attacks and the common cold, but "it is our own fault" when we contract an STD. There are preventive measures which we can use to decrease our chances of contracting the flu or STD, but placing blame helps no one and can interfere with medical and emotional care seeking behavior.

Clearly, the emotional complications of STD are an important aspect of the impact of these diseases. Including information about the emotional effect of STD in human sexuality textbooks and in courses in which STD are discussed provides a more complete representation of the total impact of these conditions. Discussing this information also may break down some of the stereotypes that exist about those people who have AIDS and other sexually transmitted diseases. Strictly clinical discussions about STD can allow participants to remain emotionally distanced from the people who contract STD and from their problems, and can, in fact, allow them to maintain their stereotyped images of these people. It is more difficult to maintain these stereotypes once presented with the much more human aspects, i.e., the emotions, involved with STD.

There are a variety of teaching methods which can be used to present information about the psychosocial impact of STD. These methods can be effective in school and community settings. It is up to the teacher or presenter to assess the particular setting and population to determine which methods would be most effective. Effective teaching may include a variety of teaching methods, sometimes flowing from one method to the other as needed by the material and students. All teaching methods should be used with clear objectives in mind to guide the teaching process. Methods should be chosen because they facilitate learning, not just because they are available, easy to use, or innovative. Also, no method is a substitute for thorough preparation by the presenter. No matter what methods you decide to use, you must be prepared. The remainder of this paper is devoted to discussing teaching methods.

LECTURES

Imparting information through lecturing can be efficient. A well-done lecture is one that is organized, based on clear learning objectives, and is not simply read to the learners (Whitman, 1982). Lecturing is appropriate when there are no other available methods to share the information. During a lecture, however, the learners are primarily passive; they are not actively involved in the learning process. The information imparted through lecture applies primarily to the lower end of the cognitive domain (knowledge) but not to the affective domain (attitude toward the subject) (Whitman & Schwenk, 1983).

However, lectures can be used to provide an important baseline of information and can be combined effectively with other teaching methods. After hearing a lecture on the psychosocial aspects of STD, students should be able to answer simple knowledge questions, relying on their ability to memorize and recall the information.

An excellent discussion of how to prepare and present lectures can be found in Whitman (1982).

AUDIOVISUALS

Audiovisuals (e.g., chalkboards, flipcharts, overhead transparencies, 35 mm slides, films, audiotapes, videotapes, filmstrips) can be effective in augmenting the information presented in a lecture format or they can serve as a trigger for starting a group discussion. If they are used as the primary source of information, the audience should be prepared beforehand. For example, before showing a videotape to a group of people, tell them what the video is about and what highlights will be presented by the video. Then they will know why they are watching it and they will listen for those important points. It also is helpful to discuss the video afterwards and to answer any questions group members might have. Presentations that combine both audio and visual stimulation are more easily remembered by audiences because these presentations require that audiences use more than one sense to experience them. As more senses become involved in the experience, the greater the probability that information will be remembered.

Cost, equipment, and availability of materials are important considerations in determining the use of audiovisuals. If you have an overhead projector, producing transparencies is relatively easy and inexpensive. Movies and videotapes, on the other hand, can be quite expensive to buy or to rent and the initial investment in equipment can be expensive. However, do not overlook some excellent opportunities for free use of materials. The American Red Cross, for example, has produced an excellent video on AIDS (*Beyond Fear*), and they make this video available without charge for use in educational programs. Also do not overlook the generosity of local television and video equipment stores. I have had very good luck in borrowing large screen televisions and video equipment from local store owners when I am presenting in local schools or other groups. It is good public relations for them and it helps you out as well.

Whenever you are going to use any commercially or professionally produced program, be sure to follow the cardinal rule of previewing the material before using it. I spoke with one junior high school teacher who was angry and upset after using a set of slides on sexually transmissible diseases. She did not preview the slides and images that shocked and embarrassed her appeared on the screen as she presented her lecture. She and her students suffered through that lecture. If you preview the material then you can decide if it is suitable for your group and if it presents material in a way that agrees with the information you wish to present. Avoid materials that present STD in a melodramatic manner (films that did this were popular when I was in high school) or materials that underestimate the maturity level of your audience. A bad film is worse than no film at all.

A more thorough discussion of audiovisuals and of their various uses can be found in Gustafson and Corcoran (1978).

GROUP DISCUSSION

Group discussions can involve learners in a much more active role than can lecturing. Group participants can contribute to the process and direction of the discussion. Group discussions also can be used to explore attitudes and to help learners to examine their own feelings about STD. It is important that group discussion participants have basic knowledge about the topic. Therefore, a discussion preceded by a lecture, by a reading assignment, or by an audiovisual presentation which provides a baseline of information about STD could be an effective teaching combination. Impetus for group discussions can come from newspaper or magazine articles, television shows, cartoons, or movies as well as many other sources.

Although group discussions do not give the leader (presenter) as much control as in a lecture situation, the leader still must be effective in maintaining control over the group. The leader has a general objective in mind and must be sure the group is working towards this objective. Well worded and well placed questions can bring the group back to the topic at hand if they stray too far. Questions directed at specific group members also can involve people who tend not to participate and can pull the discussion away from those who monopolize.

During recent presentations on AIDS, I have used student responses to scenarios as a trigger for discussion about the psychosocial aspects of AIDS. Students are given a sheet of paper which presents to them a scene in which an older brother tells the student that he (the brother) is ill. In some of the scenarios the brother has a diagnosis of AIDS, in other scenarios the diagnosis is cancer. Half of the students receive one scenario, half receive the other scenario. The students are asked to write down their reactions: verbal, emotional, and physical. After I collect the reactions, I begin to ask which scenarios the students had received. Then I ask the students who responded to the cancer scenario to describe their responses. If they are reluctant to respond, I can ask specific students specific questions about their responses—I had already asked who had which scenario. Generally, however, at least one student will begin to talk and this encourages the others to talk. I am always careful to listen to and acknowledge the responses, but not to react to them. All emotions are acceptable and taken as being real and honest. I want the students to feel free to talk. After we have heard about a range of responses and they begin to sound fairly familiar, I switch focus to the students who responded to the AIDS scenario. If these students are slow to respond, I again ask specific students specific questions to get them started. Students talk about reacting to the imaginary scenarios with anger and sadness. They also talk about confusion and a sense of loss of control. These feelings have their counterparts in the feelings experienced by people with AIDS and it is important to bring out this connection. Invariably, some students will say that their responses included fear and that this fear was based on lack of knowledge about AIDS. This response creates a good lead-in to a general discussion/lecture on AIDS. In addition, this two scenario format allows students to compare responses to two serious illnesses, one which they know they cannot catch from others (cancer) and one which many of them fear (AIDS). It also allows me to point out that at one time people reacted quite differently to people who had cancer — reactions were in many ways the same as current reactions to people with AIDS.

Gustafson and Corcoran (1978) and Whitman and Schwenk (1983) provide thorough discussions and guidelines for conducting effective group discussions.

GUEST SPEAKER/PANEL DISCUSSION

Another effective way to present information on STD is through the use of a guest speaker or several guests who make up a panel. Guest speakers have the added advantage of appearing as outside authorities on the subject and so their presentations often carry more impact than do other types of presentation. Ideally the panel would include at least one person who has been diagnosed as having an STD. This person could share his or her firsthand experiences of dealing with an STD. Obviously, it is not easy to get such a guest speaker because of the stigma already discussed. In some communities, however, there are people associated with herpes support groups or AIDS support groups who are willing to talk about what life is like for them. Other guest speakers could include those people who have counseled with persons who have STD. Many organizations establish speakers bureaus for presentations of this type.

As with other teaching methods, the audience should be prepared, it at all possible. If you are a classroom teacher, you can tell your students about the guest speaker and the topic and ask them to come to class prepared to ask a few questions. This could be turned into an assignment with points awarded for bringing to class so many written questions. When presentations are part of a community program, audience members generally self-select to come to the program and they may be prepared for the topic already. In either case, a well stated introduction can set the tone for the speaker and get the audience mentally ready. For some presentations it may be best to have audience members write down questions they might want to ask and then hand in the written questions so that they do not have to be embarrassed by being identified as being overly interested in the topic. It is not unusual for people to come up to the speaker after the presentation and after most of the audience has left so that they can ask a question in a more private atmosphere. I also have had the experience of people asking very detailed questions after a presentation and then they very quickly point out that they are simply curious, that issues of sexuality and STD really do not pertain to them personally. It would be helpful if you could arrange a period of time after a guest speaker presentation so that this type of more private exchange could take place.

ROLE PLAYING

Role playing activities are effective in presenting content in the affective domain (Gustafson & Corcoran, 1978). Participants are able to experience various roles and problem situations in a safe environment. As with other methods, participants should be prepared prior to using role playing. This preparation could involve assigned readings on STD, a lecture, or a film or video. The teacher must be prepared with written role play situations. These situations can involve a wide range of situations and variations, depending upon the participants. For example, role play could involve two people in a relationship which has evolved to the point where both partners wish to be involved sexually. One partner, however, has herpes and feels he/she must tell the other partner (Moore & Larsen, 1986). A variation could be to have both partners in a supposedly monogamous relationship when one partner is diagnosed as having herpes.

Role playing takes time but is worth that time if it is prepared well. People should not be forced into role playing because it can be embarrassing for some people to act in front of the entire group.

After the role play has gone on for about 5 minutes, stop the players and ask them to talk about what occurred during the role play. Then give the audience a chance to talk about the role play. Acting ability should not be the topic here. The audience should be instructed to speak in terms of characters' actions, and not actions of the players themselves. What should be discussed is how people felt as the characters or as the audience, what characters did and why, and what were some alternatives for the characters' actions.

As in the scenario experience described earlier, students will talk about experiencing a range of emotions during role plays. It is not unusual for the audience to experience these emotions as well. Even though they may not be directly involved, watching the role play makes the experience much more real for them. When people become deeply involved in role plays, it is not unusual for them to express their emotions by crying or yelling or being very quiet. Role plays allow participants the chance to experience these emotions more deeply than do some of the other activities. Participants may develop a better understanding of what it is like to be someone who has an STD.

Gustafson and Corcoran (1978) provide thorough guidelines for using role playing and Moore and Larsen (1986) provide role play examples specific to STD.

GUIDED IMAGERY

Guided imagery can be a powerful tool in presenting the emotional experiences related to having an STD. Through guided imagery you can set up any imaginary experience, guide the participants through the experience, and provide them the time and safe environment in which to feel the emotions related to that experience.

The ideal setting for using guided imagery is one in which participants can be comfortable and relaxed. A carpeted area where people can spread out on the floor is good, or people can be asked to bring mats or blankets. Lights should be dimmed or turned off and the room should be free from external noise. The room temperature should be neither too hot nor too cold. However, do not be discouraged and reluctant to try guided imagery if you cannot set up this ideal atmosphere. I have been in situations where participants had to sit at desk chairs, the windows let in too much light, and the much needed air conditioner made too much noise — and yet, guided imagery worked.

The beginning of any exercise of this type involves a period of relaxation. The leader uses a soft, level voice to suggest that participants focus on their breathing and to feel themselves relax with each breath:

> As you lay here on the floor, making yourself comfortable, gently closing your eyes, you may begin to notice your breath. Breathing in, breathing out. Letting your breath be full and relaxed. Letting your breath move through your whole body. You can feel your belly rise and fall with each breath. And when you next exhale, you may feel your body sinking deeper down into the floor, as you sink even deeper down inside of yourself. (Shanti Project Videotape Training Manual, 1984, p. 42)

Other relaxation techniques may be used as well. The purpose is to enable the participants to relax as much as possible and to open themselves up to the feelings they are about to experience.

Once the relaxation part of the exercise is over, guide the participants into the experience. The transition should be smooth. Guide the participants through experiencing STD symptoms, visiting a clinic, being examined and tested, hearing the diagnosis, being treated, telling sex partners about the diagnosis, and, if you are teaching about AIDS, being hospitalized and facing death. Never tell the participants what they are feeling. Let them bring that part of the experience from out of themselves. Be sure to move slowly enough through the experience that participants have time to feel the emotions that well up from inside themselves. Also be sure to move fast enough that participants do not fall asleep.

At the end of the experience, bring the participants up out of their relaxation slowly. Allow them time to "come back to the present" and to pull their thoughts together. Once people begin to sit up, open their eyes, move about and talk quietly, you can turn on the lights. Bring them together either in a large group or, if you have enough group leaders, in smaller groups to talk about their experiences and to share their feelings. For some of the participants, emotions felt during guided imagery may be very strong, the experiences may have felt real to them. They will need to talk this out, to share their anger, fear, and frustration. They will need a safe, accepting environment in which to do this. Allow people time to describe what they saw and felt. Some participants may not experience guided imagery in the same manner. They might not "see" images or the experience might not feel as real, but the experience is still valid and they need time to talk about it. Some participants will fall asleep, and you must decide if it is too disruptive to go to them to wake them up or to just let them snore. Do what is best for the group as a whole.

Doing guided imagery is a skill that needs to be practiced. If this is a group with which you will be working over a period of time, you might wish to begin doing just relaxation exercises and then work into doing short, pleasant images. Then you and the group will be prepared for a more extended, more intense guided imagery experience.

The introductory chapters of Gawain (1978) provide helpful guidelines in getting prepared to do visualization exercises. The Shanti Project Video Training Manual (1984) contains full examples of guided imagery experiences and their use.

CONCLUSION

This list and discussion of teaching methods is not meant to be exhaustive. In fact, it may be considered the tip of the iceberg of available teaching techniques. Much of what can be done is limited by the instructor's imagination. However, there are other limits to what can be done and/or discussed in various teaching situations.

Many of the barriers to education about STD stem from the same attitudes that perpetuate the stigmas attached to STD. In the school setting teachers must assess the atmosphere of the community and of the school when planning educational programs about STD. When developing new programs be sure to let the school administrators know exactly what will be going on in the classroom. They should be given a course outline, a list of objectives, copies of all handouts, and the chance to view and/or listen to any audiovisuals you plan to use. Then they will be prepared to handle any controversies which might arise. Parents also should be given the opportunity to preview this material and to request permission for their child to do some other learning activity while this information is being presented. Being open about the material being presented gives the teacher the opportunity to dispel the rumors that often accompany this type of teaching unit.

Barriers that exist in the community often come from special interest groups and sometimes from groups which are providing funding for the program. Again, openly sharing information about the program may alleviate some of the controversy. Knowing community attitudes and tailoring the program to fit the community helps break down barriers. Tailoring a program to meet the needs of a specific target group also increases the effectiveness of a program. A needs assessment is essential. A presentation on STD directed at a group of homosexual males would be quite different from a presentation on STD directed at a junior high school health class. Also, it is important to work with representatives from funding groups from the beginning of program development. A certain amount of compromise may be necessary if these groups are unhappy about parts of the program, but education about STD is important and some compromise may be worth being able to implement the program.

Reaching certain target groups also may be a barrier to education about STD. Certain segments of the population are at risk and yet getting information to them may be difficult. Educational programs about AIDS have effectively reached most of the homosexual male population in large, urban communities where there are many organizations and businesses which cater to this group. In rural areas these avenues of education and information spreading are not readily available. It is much more difficult to reach these rural gays. Educators must rely more on mass media and work at getting their programs into a wide variety of community organizations where gay men who cannot be open about their sexuality might be members. It also is difficult to reach intravenous drug users who are at risk for AIDS and hepatitis. One route of access is through drug treatment programs, but many intravenous drug users are not involved in such programs and are not readily identifiable.

There are many challenges and barriers to implementing effective educational STD programs, but education about STD and about the psychosocial impact of STD is essential in both the schools and the community. Educators who wish to address the psychosocial impact of STD must be willing to try different teaching methods which will address the attitudes and emotions of audience participants. Activities which directly involve students and encourage them to acknowledge, experience, and examine their own emotions will be most effective in teaching this aspect of STD. In this way we can teach about the entire scope of STD more effectively.

REFERENCES

Brandt, A.M. (1985). *No magic bullet: A social history of venereal disease in the United States since 1880*. New York: Oxford University Press.

Confronting AIDS. (1986). National Academy of Sciences. Washington, DC: National Academy Press.

Drob, S. (1986). Psychosexual implication of genital herpes. *Medical Aspects of Human Sexuality, 20*(8), 97, 100, 102, 104.

Gawain, S. (1978). *Creative imagery*. New York: Bantam Books.

Gustafson, M.B., & Corcoran, S.A. (1978). *Teachers' desk reference*. Ordell, NJ: Medical Economics Company.

Masters, W.H., Johnson, V.E., & Kolodny, R.C. (1986). *Masters and Johnson on sex and human loving*. Boston: Little, Brown and Company.

Moore, J.R., & Larsen, D. (1986). Sexually transmitted diseases: Role playing activities. In J.C. Orolet & J.V. Fetro (Eds.), *Instructor's resource manual for "Human Sexuality."* New York: John Wiley and Sons.

Morin, S.F., & Batchelor, W.F. (1984). Responding to the psychological crisis of AIDS. *Public Health Reports, 99*(1), 4-9.

Morin, S.F., Charles, K.A., & Malyon, A.K. (1984). The psychological impact of AIDS on gay men. *American Psychologist, 39*, 1288-1293.

Shanti Project Video Training Manual. (1984). San Francisco: Shanti Project.

Whitman, N.S. (1982). *There is no gene for good teaching: A handbook on lecturing for medical teachers*. Salt Lake City, UT: University of Utah School of Medicine.

Whitman, N.A., & Schwenk, T.L. (1983). *A handbook for group discussion leaders: Alternatives to lecturing medical students to death*. Salt Lake City, UT: University of Utah School of Medicine.

AIDS: Prevention Is the Only Vaccine Available: An AIDS Prevention Educational Program

Michael Shernoff
Luis Palacios-Jimenez

INTRODUCTION

At the time of writing over 37,386 Americans have been diagnosed with full-blown Acquired Immunodeficiency Syndrome (AIDS). (U.S. Department of Health and Human Services, 1987). Health officials estimate that for every person with AIDS, there are 10 people with AIDS Related Conditions (ARC) (San Francisco Department of Public Health, 1983). There are estimates that anywhere from one to two million Americans have already been exposed to Human Immunodeficiency Virus (HIV) (Curran, 1985; Sivak & Wormser, 1985). Thus, with an incubation rate of up to several years and with no effective vaccine, treatment or cure in sight, preventing the transmission of HIV has become the single greatest priority.

This article outlines an AIDS prevention program that the authors developed for gay and bisexual men. Concepts regarding the education of the general public are discussed, issues inherent in reaching different segments of the population are explained and finally specific suggestions for conducting effective prevention programs and their integration into practice settings are offered.

Educating the general public on lowering the risks of contracting or transmitting HIV has posed many challenges for professionals in AIDS prevention and risk-reduction efforts. Not the least of these

© 1988 by The Haworth Press, Inc. All rights reserved.

challenges is how to reach diverse segments of the general population that are at risk. Gay and bisexual men, for example are not a single homogeneous group, even when living in a major urban centre such as Manhattan or San Francisco. Some are deeply closeted or married, others have a number of concurrent sexual or romantic partners, or live in committed relationships with a single life companion or lover. Some gay men are very sophisticated sexually, while others are quite naive. Intravenous (IV) drug users, another population at risk, do not have an identified or unified community outside of residential therapeutic communities for those recovering from addiction. For some members of these two groups, sexuality and drug use may not be the major forms of identification.

Dr. Richard Keeling, Chair of the American College Health Association's Task Force on AIDS (reported in Gray, 1986) has cited a case that amply demonstrates the complexity of reaching everyone who needs AIDS prevention education. A female student who did not consider herself part of a risk group recently tested positive for HIV antibodies. She reported a three-week sexual relationship with a heterosexual male, who in turn had a two-night sexual relationship with another male. "He did not think of himself as being in a risk group and he would never define himself as gay or bisexual" Keeling says. "And that's exactly the way a lot of typically-straight males feel . . . that if it happened one or two times and it was on a camping trip and nobody knows about it . . . well then, that's not gay" (Gray, 1986, pp. 12-13).

Over the past two years, as consultants for AIDS service organizations, the authors have conducted AIDS prevention programs in the U.S. and Canada for over eight thousand people, most of whom were gay or bisexual men but some of whom were intravenous drug-using individuals or interested heterosexual women. We developed five working assumptions about doing risk reduction programs as social workers and health educators.

1. The rate and frequency of AIDS is growing.
2. AIDS is moving into all segments of the general population.
3. There is no effective treatment or cure.

4. I.V. drug users, bisexual men and heterosexually married homosexual men are the key links in the spread of AIDS into the general U.S. population.
5. AIDS is a *behaviour-bound* disease that is caused by high risk behaviours, and not by membership in particular risk groups.

AIDS can be prevented by changing behaviours. Practitioners undertaking AIDS prevention work with the general population need to discuss the specific behaviours that risk transmission of HIV — and not the risk groups. Such an approach helps to minimize the biases that affect gay or bisexual men or IV drug-using individuals, thus clearing the way to viewing AIDS and AIDS prevention as public health and not moral issues. Since contracting AIDS is behaviour bound, it is a disease with which anyone can be afflicted.

Our model for AIDS prevention education is intended to help individuals from becoming infected with HIV. We believe it can assist people to manage their lives and even their illnesses should they already have AIDS, ARC, or are HIV-antibody positive. Our model is also meant to help mental health professionals in having cognitive and affective interventions ready to use with clients that include large numbers of people at risk for contracting AIDS.

All who are at risk for AIDS should be encouraged to understand and internalize the following set of beliefs in order to promote change.

— They must recognize AIDS as a direct personal threat. Most often this occurs after someone they know has become ill or died from AIDS.
— They must understand that AIDS is preventable.
— They must work through feelings of guilt about high-risk behaviour that may have gone on before they learned how AIDS is transmitted.
— They must believe that they can learn to manage necessary lifestyle changes in order to not put themselves at risk for contracting or transmitting HIV.
— They must have peer support while undergoing these lifestyle changes.

— They must believe that they can subsequently have a satisfying
sexual and/or drug-free life (Jacobs, 1986).
— If unable to believe that they can live drug-free, then they must
believe that they can learn not to share IV drug-using para-
phernalia such as syringes and cookers and how to properly
sterilize such items between use.

PREVENTION AND TARGET POPULATIONS

Interventions geared to preventing the spread of HIV need to be
tailored to meet the specific needs of the group or individual being
addressed. People have different knowledge levels about AIDS.
While some will require basic education about specific means of
transmission, others who already have this information will only
require assistance on how to live with changes they will need to
make if they are to no longer place themselves and their sexual
partners at risk. We have adapted the tripartite model health educators use in dealing with other issues such as pregnancy and drug
abuse. This approach was tailored to address the needs of a variety
of individuals who require information about preventing the spread
of AIDS. There are three levels of prevention: primary, secondary
and tertiary.

The purpose of *primary prevention* is to prevent, reduce and delay the onset of HIV infection. There are two aspects of primary
prevention: the first consists of actions designed to prevent the development of the disease. This is a series of macro and generational
interventions. For instance the younger generation of people currently growing into sexual maturity would learn to only engage in
safer sex as a way of life until they were in a committed relationship
and both individuals tested negative for the antibodies to HIV. In
addition, the next generation of IV drug users would learn how to
use needles safely.

The second aspect of primary prevention deals with interventions
designed to promote the idea that certain life skills can assist people
in preventing exposure to HIV. For example, women who have
shared intravenous drug using implements like syringes or "cookers" or who have been the sexual partner of someone who has

shared drug using implements as well as those women whose lovers have been bisexual men, hemophiliacs or recipients of blood transfusions prior to the blood supply being screened for HIV are considered to be highly at risk for developing AIDS. Even when such high-risk women have accepted the need to use condoms, assertiveness training is one necessary component of primary prevention. Such interventions teach women how to negotiate for power and control in relationships with men who may have a history of being abusive. This is a psychosocial approach which helps people develop the necessary life skills to avoid transmission of HIV.

The goal of primary prevention is to provide information and education regarding transmission of HIV for the general population. Through this process, individuals will be enabled to determine whether they themselves may be at risk. Once this has occurred, they can be helped to substitute low-risk behaviours for those that are high-risk.

Target populations for primary prevention are: the general public, health care workers, sex educators and mental health professionals, individuals at high risk for contracting HIV and sexual partners or needle sharing partners of individuals who are at high risk.

Secondary prevention is concerned with individuals who are already positive for HIV antibodies. They may possibly be symptomatic for ARC or AIDS. The goal is to prevent them from being repeatedly exposed to HIV and from transmitting HIV.

For clinicians or educators working with this segment of the population it is important to help clients identify underlying issues. If left unexamined, these can prevent the person from believing in his or her capacity to adopt low-risk behaviours. A thought that is commonly expressed is: "I've already been exposed to HIV. So why should I bother to change my sexual or drug-using patterns?" This is best answered with the information that there is a growing body of evidence suggesting that repeated exposure to HIV may be necessary for active illness to progress.

The focus of secondary prevention is to provide information on the nature of the illness in order to retard further progression of the illness. Individuals who may be seropositive for HIV, have ARC or AIDS can learn to identify themselves so they can receive treatment and the progression and transmission of the disease can be slowed or interrupted.

Target populations for secondary prevention interventions are: individuals seropositive for HIV (these may be people who have a confirmed positive HIV antibody blood test or who simply assume seropositivity); individuals with ARC, AIDS and other HIV infections; sexual partners and needle-sharing partners of the above two groups, and members of the helping professions.

Tertiary prevention is concerned with preventing as many of the disabling aspects of AIDS as possible. Called the "Living with AIDS Model," the intent is to maximize the living potential of the person with AIDS, ARC or HIV infection. One person with AIDS explained: "You're only dying the final week of your life. Until then you're living with AIDS." Such an attitude helps prevent and manage some of the hopelessness and other transitional affective responses for the person who is ill, for their significant others and for the professional working with him or her.

Target populations for tertiary prevention are: people with progressive AIDS, ARC or HIV infection; care partners of the above group; and health care professionals involved with the ill person.

DEVELOPMENT OF THE AIDS PREVENTION PROGRAM

Prior to the onset of AIDS, workshops on Sexually Transmitted Diseases (STD) for gay men were almost non-existent until it became evident that Hepatitis B was assuming epidemic proportions in certain segments of the gay population. The AIDS epidemic in the gay and bisexual men's community created numerous crises, one of the most significant being that new sexual behaviours had to be learned in order to adapt successfully to life in the age of AIDS (Martin, 1986; McKusick et al., 1986). This was a crisis similar to other developmental crises requiring new coping behaviours and strategies in order for the individual to adapt adequately (Mandel, 1986).

AIDS service organizations, gay health care professionals and gay media each began to provide lists of what sexual behaviours were high-risk. In the early period of AIDS prevention (1982-83) the term "safer sex" had not yet been coined. Low risk sexual activity was called "healthy sex" a term itself fraught with moralistic overtones. At times information about preventing the spread of AIDS was presented in a highly-moralistic fashion. As a result, safer sex began to be viewed by some men as just another negative injunction. And in defiance of such injunctions many people refused to adopt to make peace with safer sex.

Sex and semen in particular began to be viewed as toxic. Many gay men began equating sex with death both consciously and unconsciously. It was precisely this internalized sense of toxicity which resulted in men feeling dirty, depressed and isolated. Thus many developed sex-negative or erotophobic attitudes. These attitudes easily reinforced underlying homophobic feelings, especially since some Christian fundamentalists were suggesting that AIDS was God's punishment upon homosexuals. Combined with living through an onslaught of friends and lovers dying, a general level of depression, anxiety and lowered self esteem developed among certain segments of gay men's communities around the country.

Uncertainty having to do with which sexual practices were low risk or how to change long-existing patterns of sexual behaviour contributed to this anxiety. Many men were angry about AIDS and the changes necessary to protect themselves and their sexual partners. Some felt trapped into choosing celibacy and became resentful or depressed when faced with this choice. Others felt defiant and simply refused to practice safer sex, feeling that there was no sense in having sex if they could not do whatever they wanted.

In June 1985, in response to the difficulties gay and bisexual men in New York City were reporting in adopting the risk-reduction guidelines, an AIDS-prevention workshop called "Hot, Horny and Healthy: Eroticizing Safer Sex" was developed by the authors to address these issues. Both are psychotherapists with substantial gay practices in Manhattan. As gay men who ourselves are at-risk for contracting or transmitting the AIDS virus we had to personally make the behavioural changes in our own lives that all gay and bisexual men were being asked to do. This made us sensitive to and empathetic with the difficulties inherent in being able to change one's patterns of sexual behaviour.

The workshop was developed as a sexual enrichment seminar for all gay and bisexual men whether they were single, dating or in a long-term committed relationship. It was intended for people who were healthy, as well as for those who had ARC or AIDS, and for those who were both HIV antibody positive and negative, as well as those who did not know their antibody status. It was considered important not to divide the gay community into people who were well and those who were not to help avoid the development of a caste system based on health or antibody status.

We had recognized the need to teach that safer sex could be great sex that did not have to be either dull or limited. It was considered crucial for gay and bisexual men not to give up sex because the virus thought to cause AIDS was sexually transmitted. Essentially the seminar provided the participants with the opportunity to express their feelings about changing their patterns of sexual behaviour. Through the use of large and small group exercises, discussions and role playing, participants were enabled to learn how to negotiate safer sex with a new or pre-existing partner. The participants were provided with strategies on how to make safer sex spontaneous, erotic, creative, satisfying and fun.

The workshop was different from other existing safer sex seminars insofar as it did *not* spend a great deal of time going into which behaviours were or were not high-risk. Our goal was to develop a psychoeducational model that would deal primarily with the cognitive and affective aspects of changing sexual behaviour.

It should be noted that the workshop had been originally developed for a conference sponsored by Gay Men's Health Crisis in June of 1985 and has since become an essential component of that organization's AIDS prevention programs. We have written a facilitator's guide for running the workshop so it can be replicated by others and thus not be a trainer-dependent model (Palacios & Shernoff, 1987).

WORKSHOP FORMAT

The workshop lasts between 3 and 3-1/2 hours depending upon the number of participants. Workshops have been conducted for as few as eight people and as many as four hundred at a single time. Consequently it is an inexpensive and highly-efficient macro intervention.

Yalom (1985) describes the eleven categories that help create curative factors in group therapy. While not a formal therapy group, the workshop uses such principals of group treatment to help participants achieve the desired goals of substituting low risk sexual behaviours for those that are high risk. The aspects of Yalom's theory that are especially relevant to this type of combined large and small group processes are: (1) installation of hope; (2) universality; (3) imparting of information; (4) development of socializing techniques; (5) interpersonal learning; and (6) catharsis.

The workshop is divided into four parts. The first aspect provides participants with the opportunity to express and process a variety of feelings. The focus is framed in terms of how to live as a sexually-active and sexually-responsible gay or bisexual man. The blocks to accomplishing this goal are identified. Considerable time is devoted to issues around mourning the losses of old sexual patterns. Other affective responses such as anger, sadness and boredom are elicited and dealt with during this segment.

The second part is directed towards helping people identify and understand their options. This aspect focuses on affirming that new and desirable behavioural and attitudinal changes can indeed be made. Information on a wide variety of sexual options still available is provided in small group exercises. Participation in small groups is considered important in terms of enhancing a sense of sexual possibility and adventure as well as the ability to change old patterns. Since participants work on these tasks within the context of a small ongoing work group, peer support develops which helps to create a climate of safety and fun within which these discoveries can occur.

This aspect of the workshop is also devoted to giving participants permission to explore various thoughts, feelings and actions, e.g., to be angry, sad, or relieved; to talk about sex; to miss high-risk activities; to be sexual in the face of the epidemic and to be verbally and erotically playful with a group of other men.

During the third part of the workshop we attempt to have participants integrate and accept change by discussing how to eroticize safer options. This occurs by helping participants let go of thoughts, feelings and actions that are erotophobic by providing a successful, sex positive experience in the small nonthreatening group setting. Participants often reveal that many of them entered the workshop feeling extremely negative about sex and being sexually active due to the fact that AIDS is sexually transmitted. The discussion of sexual options becomes in itself a joyful and sex-positive experience that provides an emotional foundation for participants to build upon after they leave the workshop. Thus the process undergone during the workshop itself is a metaphor for the changes we hope the participants will experience in their efforts to integrate safer sexual practices into their lives.

In the fourth part of the workshop we use role playing and values clarification exercises to help participants learn how to develop skills in negotiating safer sex agreements, maintaining these agreements and in setting limits. This increases feelings of self-confidence and thus prepares them to discuss safer sex in future encounters with potential partners.

During the first and second parts of the workshop the feelings that are most often expressed are those of anger, resentment, loss and general sex negativity. We acknowledge and validate these feelings pointing out that a lot of the men seem to be feeling similarly. By the third segment, participants begin sharing feelings of awe and disbelief that they are actually enjoying the process they are going through during the workshop. This appears to provide the hope that they can actually once again enjoy sex in an excited, enthusiastic, playful as well as safer fashion.

At the conclusion of the workshop, participants are asked, as a brief evaluative device, how their thoughts and feelings have changed as a result of their involvement. Generally, they report feeling much less anxious and depressed and more hopeful about being able to have a satisfying and risk-free sex life.

The goals of the workshop are:

1. To provide a safe and non-threatening environment in which emotionally-laden material about sex and AIDS can be explored and discussed.

2. To help gay and bisexual men identify negative affective responses induced by the AIDS crisis in relation to their sexuality and sex lives.
3. To help them work through these negative feelings in order to minimize any impairment in their psychosocial/psychosexual functioning so that low risk behaviours can be substituted for high risk ones.
4. To help participants view their reactions as appropriate responses that require new crisis-management skills.
5. To provide a structure in which participants discover and share information on how to be sexually active in low-risk ways.
6. To help participants enhance and improve levels of sexual health and functioning.
7. To help them gain practice in negotiating and contracting for safer sex.

CONCLUSIONS AND IMPLICATIONS

It should be noted that the workshop described previously is *not* an appropriate intervention for all people who are at risk for AIDS. It is effective for gay and bisexual men who have a well enough developed gay or bisexual identity to seek out gay community events. One of the difficulties with using this workshop as an effective AIDS prevention strategy for broad segments of the gay men's community is that it requires individuals to be self- motivated. People who attend are usually self-referred. Consequently very closeted gay men are less apt to come to the workshop. Therefore national campaigns stressing that safer sex is for everyone regardless of sexual orientation are sorely needed to bridge this gap. Another suggested way of reaching this group of men is to advertise workshops on safer sex in local mainstream media for all men, and specifically *not* discuss gay or bisexual issues.

There are a number of recommendations for conducting effective AIDS prevention education for the general public, for specific groups such as those comprised of women and drug users and for professionals involved in agency-based or private practice.

Information overloads should be avoided. People can only absorb so much information at any single time. It is a mistake to think that because you have an audience they must receive comprehensive information on AIDS and risk reduction at one sitting.

The message of prevention and change must be repeated over time. It should be relevant to the targeted audience. It needs to be revised when appropriate so that it speaks to women differently than to men and differently to gay and bisexual men that to IV drug-using men who may be heterosexual. A variety of strategies and interventions must be developed. The message itself as well as specific "how-tos" of changing high-risk behaviour should never be punitive. Strategies must always be empowering so that the desired behavioural and attitudinal changes can become acceptable to the person.

It should always be geared to specific behaviours, i.e., unprotected anal or vaginal intercourse, sharing needles, etc. The message should occur in a context where the targeted individuals acknowledge that a problem exists and that there is a threat to their lives.

The environment for AIDS prevention should be one where the individuals' feelings, fears and resistance are able to be identified and examined by the targeted people themselves — and not force fed to them by a trainer or clinician. The interventions should motivate the targeted groups to change their behaviours. Fear should not be used as a motivator since it cannot be sustained for this purpose for lengthy periods of time.

When attempted for a mixed audience of heterosexual men and women the participants should be segregated by sex into small groups, otherwise the men and women are not sufficiently self-revealing about their feelings and sexual tastes for the workshop to achieve the desired goals.

When conducting AIDS prevention education for women there are special issues that need to be taken into account which this workshop format is not ordinarily able to address. For women who are at high-risk a "safer sex is great sex or fun sex" approach is often not relevant since many of these women report that even prior to AIDS sex was rarely a fun or enjoyable activity for them. Realistically, some women at risk are concerned with how to begin to have their partners use condoms without creating power struggles.

There are reports of women being raped within their relationships, being battered and being threatened with the loss of the security of "a meal ticket" when they have attempted to introduce the use of condoms.

Machismo can be another barrier to implementing safer sexual practices once women have been educated about AIDS prevention. In Haitian and Hispanic male-female relationships the man is traditionally dominant and only he may introduce new ideas about sexual practices. As a result, following one seminar a woman was beaten for having suggested the idea of using a condom.

Some at risk women have reported that if their partners find condoms offensive or uncomfortable and refuse to use them, rather than leave these relationships, women stay and submit to high-risk behaviours at the risk of their own life. Therefore, teaching certain women safer sex interventions can create new and additional problems for them in their often already chaotic lives.

Other areas of resistance encountered with AIDS-prevention programs for women are religious and cultural. Many of the high-risk women are Haitian or Hispanic and may have been raised as practicing Catholics. Accordingly, the official Catholic opposition to artificial birth control is another barrier that must be taken into consideration. Thus, the special and unique issues of AIDS prevention for high-risk women still needs to be addressed, and additional interventions must be developed to meet their needs.

With regard to drug users there is a pilot program in New York City developed by a group called ADAPT (Association for Drug Abuse Prevention and Treatment) that enlists former and recovering IV drug users to educate active IV users about safer sex and safer needle use by going to parks, abandoned buildings, "shooting galleries," and other locations where addicts congregate to use or buy drugs. They also convey the message that there is treatment and cure for drug addiction currently available in New York City at methadone programs and therapeutic communities.

It is noted that active addicts are allowing the ADAPT people into the areas where drugs are being bought and used, and are engaging in conversations about AIDS and drug abuse. This approach is now being used by both the New York City Department of Health and the New York State AIDS Institute who have made funding available to hire recovered and recovering addicts and other street wise people to do this kind of AIDS prevention education.

Finally, the urgent need to insure that people reduce high risk behaviours has resulted in our introducing social health education as one aspect of our private practice. Thus, with every sexually active adult who is not in a relationship that has been monogamous for at least nine years we bring up the issue of AIDS in relation to their sexual practices. There are understandable concerns regarding the introduction of this material into treatment. Questions of whether the interview content becomes overstimulating for the client or "inappropriately eroticized" have to be weighed on a case by case basis. Many clients are not comfortable with issues of sexuality and thus may feel uncomfortable by its discussion.

For social workers in any part of North America engaged in individual, couple or group work with sexually active single adults, a newly separated or divorced person, a teenager just becoming sexually active, or any gay or bisexual man, it becomes appropriate to ask: "How do you feel about the fact that AIDS is sexually transmitted?" and "What are you doing to protect yourself from becoming infected?" These kinds of questions can raise many feelings including intense anger. These arise most often because any discussion of the subject shatters the client's denial that AIDS cannot touch him or her. The anger can also often emerge when the client perceives the question itself as a parental negative injunction. Negative transferential feelings that arise provide fertile ground for exploration of a variety of related issues like taking care of one's self, self image, the consequences of impulsive behaviour as well as an examination of the transference itself.

When anger or shock dissipates, asking clients to explore how they might need to change their sexual practices can be fruitful. Feelings about condoms, and what can be done to eroticize their use need to be explored. The authors have worked with clients who have become sexually abstinent in response to AIDS. Following initially successful experiences using condoms on a date, these clients often immediately began a phase of treatment where there was an idealized transference towards the therapist as a result of resumption of sexual activity. Ultimately, this has to be worked through for treatment to progress.

We have asked clients to imagine specific sensate focus exercises where they touch or are being touched by a sexual partner in ways that will not put either of them at risk. It is not necessary that the specifics of what these acts are to be verbalized to the therapist. Similarly, the therapist can ask the client to imagine safer ways of doing a variety of sexual practices. Having a client role play how to initiate a conversation about safer sex during a session has also proven to be a helpful exercise. Clients have reported that these exercises proved helpful in improving the quality of their sex lives since it taught them how to better focus on their own sexual needs and wants as well as those of their partner.

In summary, a format and process for providing AIDS prevention education for the general population has been outlined. A particular approach that has been useful in addressing the needs of openly gay and bisexual men has been detailed as an example. Given the confines of the current conservative political environment we note the challenge inherent in how to proclaim the message that prevention is the only vaccine available for AIDS.

REFERENCES

Curran, J. et al. (1985). The epidemiology of AIDS: Current status and future prospects. *Science,* 229: 1352-1357.

Grey, John. (1986). Colleges, students, and AIDS: A new awareness. *New York Native,* Issue 184, 12-13.

Jacobs, Raymond. (1986). Closing remarks, public health session 18. *Proceedings of the International Conference on Acquired Immune Deficiency Syndrome,* Paris, France.

Mandel, Jeffrey. (1986). The psychosocial challenges of AIDS and ARC. *Focus: A Review of AIDS Research,* Jan.

Martin, John L. (1986). Sexual behavior patterns, behavior change, and occurrence of antibody to LAV/HTLVIII among New York City gay men. *International Conference on AIDS,* Paris, France, June.

McKusick, Leon et al. (1986). Reported changes in the sexual behavior of men at risk for AIDS San Francisco 1982-1984, the AIDS research project. *Public Health Reports.*

Palacios-Jimenez, Luis & Shernoff, Michael. (1987). *A facilitator's guide to eroticizing safer sex, a psychoeducational workshop approach to safer sex education.* Gay Men's Health Crisis.

San Francisco Department of Public Health. (1983). *AIDS activity office: AIDS mental health proposal.* (Unpublished).

Sivak, S.L. & Wormser, G.P. (1985). How common is HTLVIII infection in the
    United States? *New England Journal of Medicine,* v, 313:1352.
United States Department of Health and Human Services. (1987). Public Health
    Service. Centre for Disease Control. *Morbidity and mortality weekly report,*
    June 15.
Yalom, Irvin. (1975). *The theory and practice of group psychotherapy.* New
    York: Basic Books.

PART IV: EPILOGUE

The Approaching Epidemic

Allan Brandt

The AIDS epidemic has — in the last five years — brought sexually transmitted diseases to the centre of medical and social consciousness once again. Not since the early twentieth century has there been such concern about the nature and impact of sexually transmitted infection. And indeed, not since the world-wide pandemic of swine influenza of 1918 have we faced a public health emergency of such tragic magnitude. In this respect we have few models for approaching the AIDS epidemic. For societies that believed that epidemic infectious diseases were problems for the developing world or historians, AIDS is a painful reminder of our biomedical hubris. The epidemic is staggering in its dimensions. According to the World Health Organization as many as 100 million individuals around the globe are expected to be infected with human immunodeficiency virus (HIV) by 1991. As this issue of *Journal of Social Work & Human Sexuality* makes clear, no aspect of modern society will remain untouched in the wake of this crisis. No social work practice can avoid its repercussions. Immediate work is required to assure that our responses are rational, constructive, and humane.

Disease, of course, is not merely a biological phenomena; it is

© 1988 by The Haworth Press, Inc. All rights reserved.   *151*

shaped by powerful social, cultural, and behavioural forces. As the essays in this volume have elucidated, only a recognition of the full complex of variables shaping patterns of disease will permit us to address them in an effective and just manner. Our response to the AIDS epidemic will, no doubt, reveal our deepest values and beliefs. The epidemic will test not only our professions, our health care systems but our social institutions as well.

The social work profession, characterized by a particular, historical set of skills and sensitivities, may play a critically important role in shaping responses to the epidemic. As the articles in this volume point out, in the realms of clinical services, education, research, and public policy, social work offers a significant component of a comprehensive approach to the epidemic. Moreover, in the twentieth century, social workers have been among the leaders in the battles against sexually transmitted infections. Indeed, AIDS raises—with greater immediacy—a series of problems that health professionals have long recognized when addressing STD. We know, for example, that the traditional stigmatization of victims merely encourages denial, isolation, and perhaps further transmission of infections. We know the psychological implications of victim-blaming. We know that compulsory public health measures have generally failed to control sexually transmitted diseases. And we know that medical rather than moral approaches offer the best chance of success from both a clinical and a public health perspective.

Nevertheless, at a moment in time when *one* sexually transmitted disease is potentially lethal, it is important to avoid grouping these diseases together. Although much about AIDS is in fact similar to other STD, as a sociocultural phenomena, it is profoundly different. AIDS' high mortality among the young, and the deep fears it has generated, make it unique. Unlike other important contemporary STD, AIDS is a truly catastrophic disease with enormous social implications.

Social work may serve not only the victims of HIV infection, assisting them with the difficult psychosocial ramifications of disease. It may serve the general social good through education, prevention, and risk reduction. As the articles in this collection make clear, for every patient there is a significant constellation of lovers, family, and friends. This is important not only for assuring no further transmission of disease, but for dealing with the concerns, fears, and grief that may surround the victims of disease. The social dimension of sexually transmitted disease means that the repercussions cannot be limited to those who become infected. Broader educational programs must ultimately prepare us to cope with the inevitable uncertainties of life during an epidemic.

Social workers and other health care workers must realize that in the current health crisis our ability to construct healthy sexual attitudes and values may be seriously impaired. We sit on the edge of an era that could easily become characterized by a sexual hysteria with severe psychosocial morbidity. A second epidemic in which fear and loathing concerning all sexuality remains a serious possibility. Social workers are in a unique position through the provision of education, counseling, and supportive services to prevent this epidemic. Health care professionals must work to define the nature of healthy sexuality in a time when sexual practices hold new risks. In this respect, the necessity for a full assessment of one's own sexual values, beliefs, and attitudes will be critical for professionals if they are to be able to deal compassionately and effectively with their patients.

Because health professionals must provide such critical services in the current health crisis, we must assess the nature of the working environment and the demands placed upon them. Even in these brief, early years of the epidemic, issues of stress, coping, and emotional burn-out are already widely recognized among those who have devoted significant aspects of their practices to the care of AIDS patients. Given the most conservative estimates of future infection and disease, the demands on health care systems will be massive. We must, therefore, consider not only the costs in health dollars, but the vast human resources required. Most importantly, methods for training and sustaining health care workers in obviously difficult and stressful work must be researched and implemented. We will need to learn to care adequately for the care-givers.

While biomedical solutions offer much hope, there will be no single "magic bullet." Yet even without a "therapeutic fix," the AIDS crisis can be mitigated. More creative and sophisticated approaches are required. Recognizing that behavioural changes may be a significant factor in disease, new techniques to assist those who seek to change are required. We need to recognize that behavioural change does not mean encouraging celibacy, heterosexuality, or "morality," by anyone's definition; it means developing ways to avoid coming into contact with a deadly pathogen.

The social costs of ineffective, draconian public health measures would only augment the crisis we know as AIDS. In the context of fear that surrounds AIDS, there is a clear potential for policies which despite having little or no potential for slowing the epidemic could have considerable legal, social, and cultural appeal. The high morality associated with AIDS and the growing number of cases could become the justification for drastic measures. "Better safe than sorry" could well become a catch phrase to justify dramatic abuses of human rights in the context of an uncertain science. Moreover, the social construction of this disease, its close association in much of the public's eye with violations of the moral code could contribute to spiralling hysteria and anger which has already led to further victimization of victims, the double jeopardy of lethal disease and social oppression. This will be avoided only if we are adept in both our medical and our cultural understanding of the disease. Social work may play a critical role in the public process of discerning irrational fear from appropriate concern.

A generation from now we may look back at the AIDS epidemic proud of the way our civilization responded to a fundamental biological threat; or, we may look back marking the epidemic as the initial force that exacerbated the deepest and bitterest divisions that characterize our world. Only if we are sophisticated in our understanding of the powerful psychological, social and cultural forces which will shape our response may we assure that we address the crisis effectively, humanely, and compassionately. Social workers have both the responsibility and the opportunity to serve in the vanguard of this effort.

Index

Abortion, 28
Acquired immune deficiency syndrome
   (AIDS), 16-18,55
  asymptomatic, 39,41,48
  in bisexuals, 38
    children of, 72,80,81-82
    spouses of, 72,80-82
  causal virus. *See* Human
    immunodeficiency virus (HIV)
  in children, 41,46
  dementia related to, 18,109
  educational curricula regarding, 106-115,
    135-50
    children, 109-110
    curricula elements, 107-113
    ethical content, 109
    ethnic-racial minority groups, 110,111
    evaluation of, 113-114
    family, 109
    format, 106-107
    heterosexual at-risk groups, 110-111
    intravenous drug users, 110
    prevention, 111-112,135-150
    psychiatric complications, 108-109
    sociopsychological complications,
      108-109,125,126-127,130,132
    theory of, 106-107
    workplace issues, 112
  emotional responses to, 76,108-109,122
  as epidemic, 151-154
  first report of, 7,40,17
  geographical point of origin, 40-41
  government policies towards, 42,45-46
  as heterosexual disease, 41
  high risk groups, 17,38
  homosexual/lesbian community response,
    82-85
  in homosexuals, 42-51

  families of, 72,74-75,76-80
  homophobic response, 43,45,47,49,83
  lovers' response, 72,73-75
  prevention, 47-48,51
  prevention programs, 135-150
  hospital costs, 37,38
  incidence, 17,37,38-39,135
  HIV antibody positive diagnosis and, 1
  projected, 37,71
  worldwide, 40-41
  incubation time, 37
  in minority groups, 42-53
    behavioral effects, 47-48
    incidence, 43-44
    psychological effects, 47
    racism and, 45,49
    social work practice implications, 39,
      48-51
  mortality rate, 38
    projected, 37,71
  natural history of, 39-41
  opportunistic illness of, 18,37-38
  prevention, 18
    therapist's role in, 148-149
  prevention-related educational programs,
    111-112,135-150
    behavioral change beliefs, 137-138
    for drug addicts, 136,138-139,140,
      146,147-148
    homophobia and, 141
    primary prevention, 138-139
    safe-sex approach, 140-142,143-144,
      145,146-149
    secondary prevention, 139-140
    target populations, 138-140
    tertiary prevention, 140
    for women, 136,138-139,146-147,148
  prognosis, 37,38

© 1988 by The Haworth Press, Inc. All rights reserved.

Printed and bound by CPI Group (UK) Ltd, Croydon, CR0 4YY

17/10/2024

01775687-0016